AT HOME SOMATIC THERAPY EXERCISES FOR BEGINNERS

EASY & GENTLE MOVEMENTS FOR NERVOUS SYSTEM REGULATION EMOTIONAL HEALING, AND LASTING CALM

S.C. MONROE

DISCLAIMER

This book is intended for educational and informational purposes only. It is not a substitute for professional medical advice, diagnosis, or treatment. The practices described are general, gentle, body-awareness exercises intended to support relaxation, self-regulation, and mindful movement.

Always listen to your body and proceed at your own pace. If you have a medical condition or concerns about your physical or mental health, consult a qualified healthcare professional before beginning any new movement practice.

The author does not claim to diagnose, treat, cure, or prevent any medical or psychological condition.

CONTENTS

INTRODUCTION

Chronic pain, tension, and stress have become all too common in our fast-paced, modern lives. A staggering 77% of adults report experiencing physical symptoms caused by stress, while over 50 million Americans struggle with chronic pain. These challenges can leave us trapped, limited, and desperate for relief. But what if I told you there's a way to break free from this cycle of discomfort and reclaim your well-being?

Enter somatic exercises—a gentle yet powerful approach to healing that focuses on regulating the nervous system and relieving stress through intentional movement. Unlike traditional forms of exercise that prioritize pushing your body to its limits, somatic exercises emphasize listening to your body's wisdom and working with it to release deeply held tension.

In this book, I aim to make somatic exercises accessible to everyone, regardless of age, fitness level, or experience. By sharing the science behind these practices and providing step-by-step guidance, I aim to shift the perception of somatic exercises from a niche therapy to a mainstream tool for physical and emotional well-being.

As you incorporate somatic exercises into your daily life, you can expect to experience many benefits. Enhanced body awareness will help you identify and address areas of tension before they become chronic issues. Reduced muscle tightness and pain will allow you to move more quickly and flexibly. Improved nervous system regulation will lead to lower stress levels, better sleep, and a greater sense of overall balance.

I understand that you may feel skeptical or overwhelmed, especially if you've tried countless other approaches without success. But I want you to know this book is designed specifically for your needs. Whether you're a complete beginner or have some experience with somatic practices, you'll find clear, actionable guidance that meets you where you are.

Throughout these pages, we'll journey from the foundational concepts of somatic exercises to more advanced techniques. Each chapter builds upon the last, ensuring you have a solid understanding of the principles and providing numerous opportunities to practice and integrate the exercises into your daily life.

As you embark on this healing path, I encourage you to approach the process with curiosity, patience, and self-compassion. Celebrate your small victories and trust that, with consistent practice, you'll experience the transformative power of somatic exercises firsthand.

So, are you ready to unlock your body's natural capacity for healing and resilience? To experience greater flexibility, less pain, and a profound mind-body connection? Then, let's dive in together and discover how somatic exercises can revolutionize your well-being, one gentle movement at a time.

CHAPTER 1

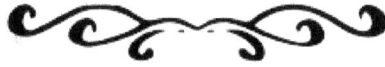

UNDERSTANDING THE FOUNDATIONS OF SOMATIC EXERCISES

You stand at a crossroads, caught between the demands of life and your body's quiet pleas for attention. Have you ever wondered why, after a stressful day, your shoulders feel like they're carrying the weight of the world? Or why your mind races at night, refusing to let you rest? These everyday experiences reflect a deeper connection between your body and mind—a connection that Somatic Therapy Exercises can help you tap into.

Somatic Therapy Exercises offer a fresh perspective on movement and wellness. They are more than just physical activity. They focus on how your body and brain communicate and how this communication affects your well-being. Unlike traditional exercises, which often emphasize strength and endurance, Somatic Therapy Exercises prioritize nervous system regulation and stress relief. They help you become aware of how you move and feel, which can lead to profound changes in both body and mind.

The goal of this book is simple: to make Somatic Therapy Exercises accessible to you. Whether you're dealing with stiffness, stress, or want to feel more at peace with yourself, this book is here to guide you. You will find practical exercises and insights that can easily fit into your daily routine. With Somatic Therapy Exercises, you can improve flexibility, reduce chronic tension, and enhance your emotional well-being.

This chapter sets the stage by explaining the science behind Somatic Therapy Exercises. Understanding these foundations will empower you to use these practices effectively. From the basics of how your nervous system works to the benefits of regular practice, you'll learn how Somatic Therapy Exercises can be a vital part of your self-care.

1.1 THE SCIENCE OF SOMATIC THERAPY EXERCISES: BRIDGING BODY AND MIND

When you move, your brain and body engage in a constant dialogue. This ongoing conversation involves feedback loops that help regulate your actions and reactions. Somatic Therapy Exercises tap into these loops to promote healing. At the heart of this process is neurophysiology, the science of how the brain and nervous system interact with the body. By understanding this connection, you can see how Somatic Therapy Exercises help manage stress and improve overall health.

One key aspect of Somatic Therapy Exercises is proprioception. Proprioception is your body's ability to sense its position and movement in space. It acts like an internal GPS, guiding your movements and helping you stay balanced. When you practice Somatic Therapy Exercises, you refine this sense of awareness. It becomes sharper, allowing you to move with more understanding and control. This heightened awareness helps reduce the risk of injury and enhances your body's ability to heal.

Physically, these exercises offer many benefits. Regular practice can help lower cortisol levels, the hormone associated with stress. When cortisol levels drop, you feel calmer and less anxious. Your muscles also become more coordinated, and your flexibility increases. This means you can move with greater ease and confidence. Over time, you might notice an increased range of motion, allowing you to perform daily tasks with less effort.

Psychologically, the benefits of Somatic Therapy Exercises are profound and multifaceted. Engaging in these practices, individuals often experience a notable decrease in symptoms associated with anxiety and depression. This improvement stems from the exercises' ability to fine-tune the nervous system, fostering a sense of serenity and heightened concentration. Regular practice allows you to cultivate an acute mindfulness of your physical state and its intricate needs. This heightened bodily awareness ushers in improved emotional regulation. As you develop this skill, you equip yourself with the tools to navigate stress more effectively, transforming your reactions from impulsive responses to considered actions. This evolution in how you perceive and interact with your emotional landscape is instrumental in cultivating a resilient and balanced mental state. Somatic Therapy Exercises adopt a holistic approach, recognizing the links between physical and psychological health. Integrating mind-body practices, such as meditation, engages both your body and mind in a healing process. This approach encourages you to listen to your body's signals, fostering a deeper connection between your physical sensations and emotional experiences.

As you explore Somatic Therapy Exercises, you will notice these shifts in how you feel and move. The benefits extend beyond physical changes. They address aspects of your life that traditional exercise routines often overlook. This chapter provides the foundation for understanding and appreciating these transformative practices.

1.2 KEY PRINCIPLES: AWARENESS, BREATH, AND MOVEMENT

Awareness forms the foundation of Somatic Therapy Exercises. It acts as a guiding light, helping you to understand your body's needs and signals more effectively. By developing this awareness, you tune into the subtle cues your body communicates. This is crucial for effective practice. Imagine you are at your desk and feel a creeping tension in your neck. You might ignore it on a busy day, but with heightened awareness, you notice it. Adjust your posture, stretch gently, and prevent it from becoming a headache. Such small interventions can make a big difference. Techniques to enhance this awareness include simple mindfulness practices. Begin by sitting quietly, noticing your breath, and then scan your body for any areas of tension or discomfort. With practice, you learn to identify these signals early and respond thoughtfully before they escalate into pain or stress.

Breath serves as a bridge between the mind and body. It plays a vital role in supporting the effects of somatic exercises. Controlled breathing can soothe the nervous system, promoting calmness and focus. When you feel anxious, your breath often becomes shallow. By taking slow, deep breaths, you signal your body to relax. This technique is effective for reducing stress and enhancing concentration. In Somatic Therapy Exercises, breath harmonizes with movement. As you move, you breathe in a way that supports each action. This might mean inhaling deeply as you stretch upward and exhaling as you fold forward. This synchronization enhances the movement, making it more fluid and effective. It also encourages a state of mindfulness, where your attention is fully present in the moment.

Movement in Somatic Therapy Exercises is not about pushing through pain or achieving a specific outcome; it's about cultivating a deeper understanding of the body. It's about exploring how your body moves naturally and finding patterns that feel good. These movements often resemble gentle, flowing motions. They might remind you of tai chi or soft yoga flows. Engaging in these movements facilitates change and healing within your body. You encourage your muscles to relax and your joints to become more flexible. Over time, these patterns help regulate your nervous system. They teach your body to respond to stress with more ease and resilience.

Together, awareness, breath, and movement create a powerful synergy. They work in harmony to unlock the benefits of Somatic Therapy Exercises. Consider the experience of a teacher who introduced Somatic Therapy Exercises in her classroom. She noticed her students, often restless and unfocused, could benefit from some calm. She led them through a simple exercise where they focused on breathing while slowly moving their arms in a circle. The room grew quiet as the students settled into the lesson's rhythm. They became more attentive and engaged in their lessons afterward. This example showcases how the elements of Somatic Therapy Exercises can work together to create a more balanced state of mind and body.

1.3 OVERCOMING COMMON MISCONCEPTIONS AND OBJECTIONS

Many people believe Somatic Therapy Exercises are only for advanced practitioners. They see the term "somatic" and think it requires specialized knowledge or a high level of fitness. But this isn't true. Somatic Therapy Exercises are designed for everyone. They are simple and adaptable, making them suitable for all ages and abilities. You don't need to be flexible or strong to start. You only need the willingness to listen to your body and follow its lead. Unlike some workouts that push you to your limits, Somatic Therapy Exercises invite you to explore your own pace and rhythm. They encourage understanding your own body's needs and responses. This approach makes them accessible to anyone willing to try. Beginners often find these exercises approachable, with many sharing positive experiences after just a few sessions. These exercises don't demand more than what you're ready to give. They meet you exactly where you are.

Another common misconception is that Somatic Therapy Exercises are equivalent to other mind-body practices. While they share some similarities, such as promoting relaxation and awareness, Somatic Therapy Exercises stand apart in their specific focus. They aim to connect movement with the nervous system, promoting balance and reducing stress. Many mind-body practices focus on maintaining proper posture and alignment. Somatic Therapy Exercises focus on how movements feel and their impact on overall well-being. This focus on internal experience rather than external form makes Somatic Therapy Exercises unique and compelling. They work from the inside out, helping you feel more at ease in your skin.

Some people question the effectiveness of Somatic Therapy Exercises. They wonder if such gentle movements can truly offer benefits. However, research supports their value. Studies have shown that these exercises can lead to significant improvements in both physical and emotional health. Evidence from neuroscience highlights how these exercises can help regulate your body's stress response. They can also improve mood and enhance emotional stability. By practicing them regularly, you can experience these benefits firsthand. You can relieve tension and stress without intense or strenuous activity. These exercises prove that sometimes, less is more.

While sometimes perceived as niche or reserved for specialized therapeutic contexts, Somatic Therapy Exercises are grounded in scientific principles and have earned a place within the broader spectrum of mainstream wellness practices. This misconception likely stems from a lack of widespread awareness about the versatility and profound benefits these exercises offer. Far from being just another trend, Somatic Therapy Exercises are a practical and effective approach for managing stress and promoting overall well-being. Their simplicity belies their power; gentle, mindful movements complement other health and wellness practices, enriching one's wellness journey rather than complicating it. Traditional exercise regimes often prioritize physical outcomes—such as muscle strength, endurance, and weight loss—with less emphasis on the mental and emotional benefits.

In contrast, Somatic Therapy Exercises offer a holistic pathway to well-being, emphasizing the interconnection between physical health and mental resilience. This approach does not replace other forms of physical activity; instead, it enhances them. By incorporating somatic practices into your daily routine, you can achieve a more balanced and comprehensive approach to your overall well-being. These exercises are designed to fit seamlessly into any lifestyle, supporting and amplifying the benefits of existing exercise routines without necessitating the abandonment of those activities. Moreover, the adaptability of Somatic Therapy Exercises means they can be easily incorporated into various parts of your day, whether it's a morning routine to awaken the body, a midday series to reset and focus, or an evening practice to unwind and de-stress. This flexibility ensures that Somatic Therapy Exercises are a valuable addition to your wellness toolkit, a sustainable, and enjoyable part of your daily life.

Through regular practice, you can cultivate a deeper connection to your body, resulting in significant improvements in stress management, emotional balance, and overall physical well-being. Consider the experience of someone who tried traditional exercise for stress relief but found it lacking. They switched to Somatic Therapy Exercises and noticed a big difference. The gentle movements helped them relax and feel more connected to their body. They found that these exercises fit easily into their day at home or work. This shift in approach brought about a newfound sense of well-being. This person isn't alone. Increasing numbers of people are discovering the benefits of somatic exercises and how they can enrich their lives.

In essence, Somatic Therapy Exercises offer a fresh perspective on wellness. They invite you to explore how your body moves and feels in a way that promotes healing. They are accessible, practical, and grounded in science. They offer a simple yet profound approach to enhancing your quality of life. By embracing them, you can learn to move and feel more at ease.

1.4 THE ROLE OF NEUROPLASTICITY IN SOMATIC PRACTICES

Imagine your brain as a flexible, ever-changing landscape. This ability to adapt and change is called neuroplasticity. It's the brain's way of reorganizing itself by forming new connections between neurons. These changes occur in response to new experiences, learning, or injury. Neuroplasticity enables you to acquire new skills, recover from setbacks, and adapt to environmental changes. It's a vital process that supports growth and healing. In the context of Somatic Therapy Exercises, neuroplasticity plays a central role. These exercises help your brain form new neural pathways. This process enhances the communication between your body and mind.

Somatic Therapy Exercises provide a unique approach to promoting neuroplasticity. As you engage in these practices, you create new neural pathways that enhance motor learning and coordination. This means your brain becomes better at coordinating your movements. With practice, movements become smoother, and your body learns to respond more efficiently and precisely. This happens because the brain's map of your body becomes clearer. You become more aware of how you move and feel. This awareness helps you refine your actions, making them more efficient.

Improved neuroplasticity leads to lasting benefits. Over time, you notice sustained improvements in how you move. Your body feels more in sync with your mind. This harmony makes everyday tasks seem easier and less taxing. Climbing stairs, bending down, or lifting objects requires less effort. These changes extend beyond physical abilities. Enhanced neuroplasticity also supports long-term emotional resilience. You become better equipped to handle stress and emotional challenges. Your brain learns to process emotions more healthily, reducing the impact of negative experiences.

Real-world examples show the power of neuroplasticity in action. Consider the story of a person who struggled with chronic pain for years. Traditional treatments offered little relief. They turned to Somatic Therapy Exercises as a last resort. With time and practice, they noticed significant changes. Their pain levels decreased, and their mobility improved. They became more confident in their movements. This person experienced a transformation that went beyond physical healing. They gained a sense of control over their body and emotions. This story illustrates how neuroplasticity can lead to profound change.

Neuroplasticity makes Somatic Therapy Exercises a powerful tool for personal growth. These exercises tap into the brain's natural ability to adapt and enhance its performance. They encourage a deeper connection between body and mind, promoting healing on multiple levels. As you practice, you engage in a process that strengthens your brain's ability to form new patterns. These patterns support both physical and emotional well-being. They enable you to navigate life with greater ease and resilience.

Incorporating Somatic Therapy Exercises into your daily routine is key to unlocking the vast potential of neuroplasticity. These practices pave the way for personal growth and healing, opening a gateway to a markedly improved quality of life. By actively engaging in Somatic Therapy Exercises, you stimulate the development of new neural connections within your brain. This, in turn, significantly enhances your brain's ability to adapt to a wide range of challenges—whether physical, emotional, or cognitive. Such adaptability is instrumental in promoting a healthier, more harmonious existence, harmonizing the dynamic relationship between body and mind. As you commit to a regular practice of Somatic Therapy Exercises, you embark on a transformative journey that leverages the power of neuroplasticity. This journey involves creating robust neural pathways that facilitate a seamless flow of communication between your nervous system and bodily movements. Over time, this enhanced neural communication supports physical agility and ease, emotional resilience, and well-being. The profound changes that ensue are not instantaneous but evolve gradually, reflecting the cumulative effect of your dedication and practice. Embracing somatic exercises as a part of your lifestyle equips you with the tools to navigate life's challenges with greater ease and resilience. The adaptability fostered through these practices ensures a balanced and healthy existence, setting the stage for continuous improvement and self-discovery. Consequently, the positive effects of neuroplasticity become tangible, manifesting as noticeable enhancements in your physical mobility, emotional stability, and overall quality of life. Thus, by dedicating time and effort to somatic exercises, you actively shape the desired changes, bringing them within your reach.

1.5 HOW SOMATIC THERAPY EXERCISES DIFFER FROM TRADITIONAL WORKOUTS

Many people are familiar with traditional forms of exercise. These often focus on external achievements, such as building muscle, losing weight, or improving endurance. In contrast, Somatic Therapy Exercises shift the focus inward. They emphasize internal awareness over external performance. This means you listen to your body's signals rather than pushing it to meet a specific goal. You should focus on lifting weights or running faster in a typical gym setting. However, with Somatic Therapy Exercises, the aim is to understand how your body feels and responds. You pay attention to subtle sensations, which can lead to profound changes in your movement and emotional state.

Somatic Therapy Exercises also prioritize regulating the nervous system, which differs from traditional workouts that primarily aim for physical fitness. Somatic practices seek to calm and balance your body's stress responses. They focus on reducing tension and promoting relaxation, which can lead to a more peaceful state of mind. For example, while lifting weights or running might increase your heart rate and adrenaline, Somatic Therapy Exercises encourage deep breathing and gentle movements. This approach helps your body find its natural rhythm, which can improve overall health and well-being.

The goals of these two exercise types also differ. Traditional workouts often focus on developing strength and endurance. You might aim to lift a certain weight or run a certain distance. In contrast, Somatic Therapy Exercises focus on promoting well-being and reducing stress. The goal is to feel better, both physically and emotionally. These exercises recognize that the mind and body are connected. By moving with awareness, stress melts away, and you feel more centered. This holistic approach can lead to improvements in mood and mental clarity.

Somatic Therapy Exercises offer unique benefits that traditional workouts might not. One advantage is the potential for improvements in emotional and mental health. The gentle and mindful nature of these exercises can reduce feelings of anxiety and depression. They encourage you to slow down and tune in to your body's needs. This can lead to increased mindfulness and emotional stability. Another benefit is the emphasis on personalization and adaptability. Somatic Therapy Exercises can be tailored to fit your unique needs and abilities. You don't need to follow a strict routine or meet specific targets. Instead, you can adapt the exercises to suit your particular situation, whether you're recovering from an injury or just beginning your fitness journey.

Consider the experience of someone who transitioned from traditional workouts to Somatic Therapy Exercises. They had spent years lifting weights and running, but still felt tense and stressed. After trying Somatic Therapy Exercises, they noticed a shift. The gentle movements helped them relax and feel more connected to their body. They found that these exercises fit easily into their daily routine and left them feeling refreshed and calm. This personal story highlights the difference between the two approaches. It shows how Somatic Therapy Exercises can offer benefits beyond physical fitness.

In summary, Somatic Therapy Exercises present a different path to wellness. They encourage you to focus on your feelings rather than what you achieve. By prioritizing internal awareness and nervous system regulation, they offer a holistic approach to health. This can lead to improvements in both physical and emotional well-being. Whether you're seeking an alternative to traditional workouts or a way to manage stress, Somatic Therapy Exercises offer a gentle and effective option. You can find balance and peace in your everyday life through mindful movement and a focus on your body's needs.

Somatic Neck release (seated)

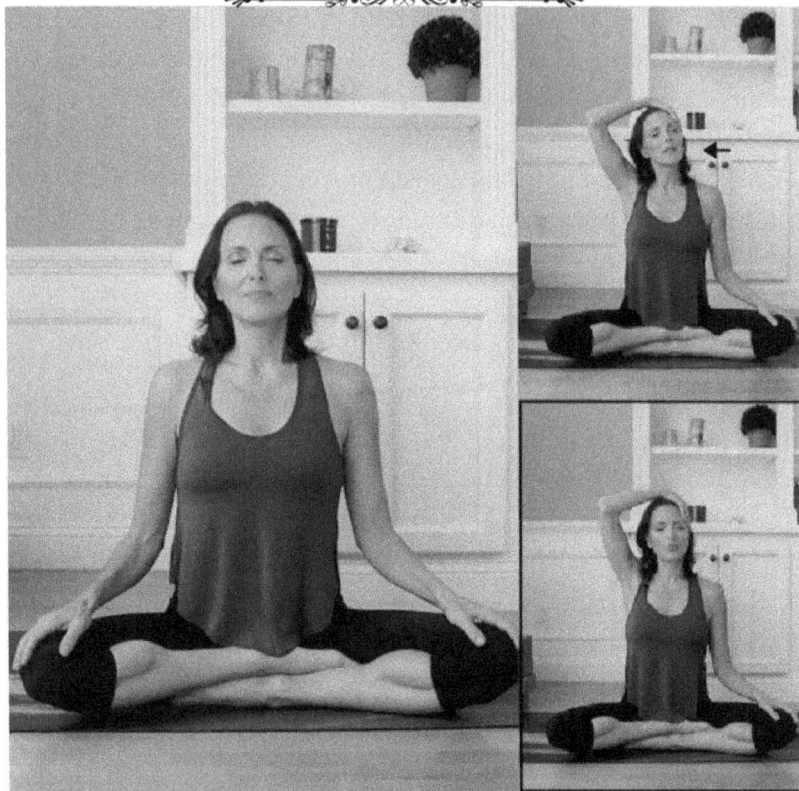

- Sit comfortably in a cross-legged position (or on a chair if needed), keeping your spine tall and shoulders relaxed.

- Place your right hand gently on the left side of your head, and let your left hand rest beside you or on your thigh.

- Take a deep breath to center yourself and prepare for mindful movement.

- On an exhale, gently tilt your head to the right, bringing your right ear closer to your right shoulder.

- Avoid pulling or forcing the stretch—let gravity and breath guide the release.

- Keep your shoulders soft and your jaw relaxed.

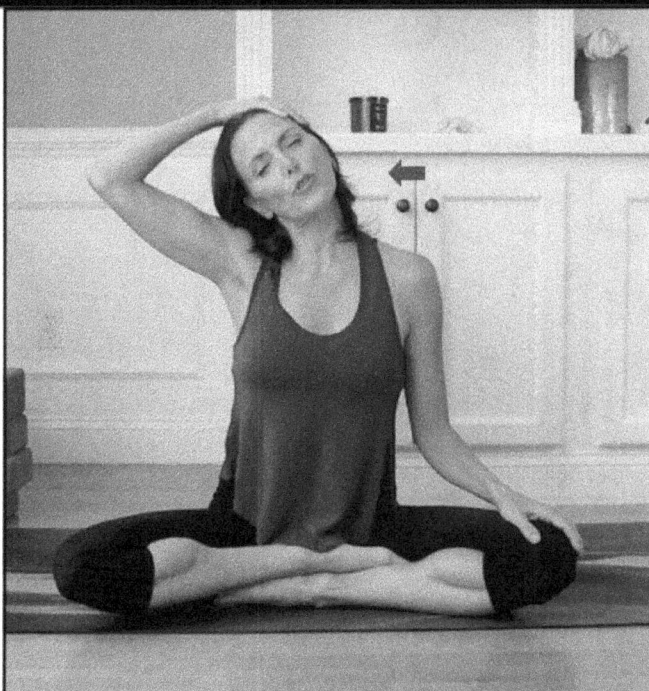

- Hold the position for 10-15 seconds while breathing deeply.

- On each exhale, allow your neck muscles to soften and your head to sink slightly deeper if comfortable.

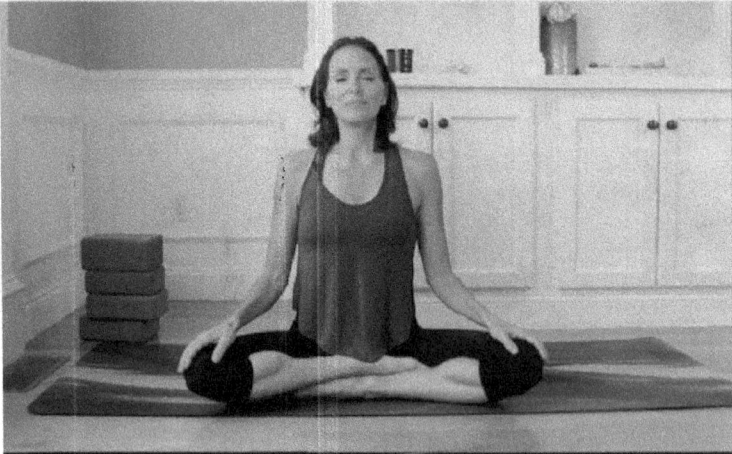

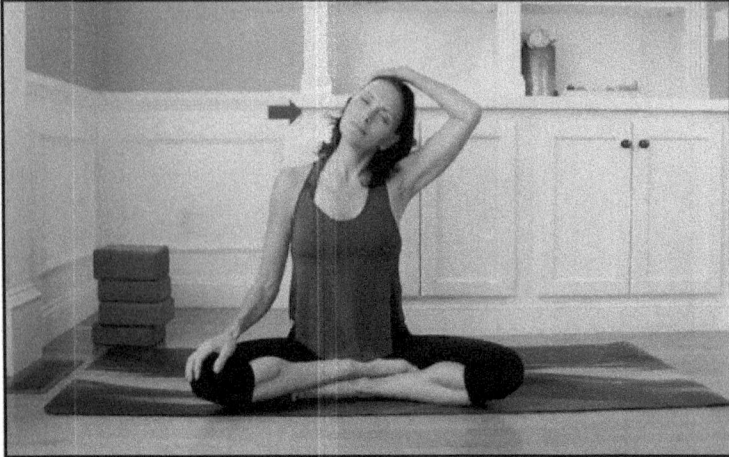

- Inhale as you slowly bring your head back to center.

- Switch sides by placing your left hand on the right side of your head and repeat the same process to the left.

- Perform 2-3 slow rounds per side, focusing on sensation, breath, and release, not on stretch intensity.

Somatic Shoulder Circles

- Lie on your back with knees bent.

- Place your hand on your shoulder, elbow pointing upward.

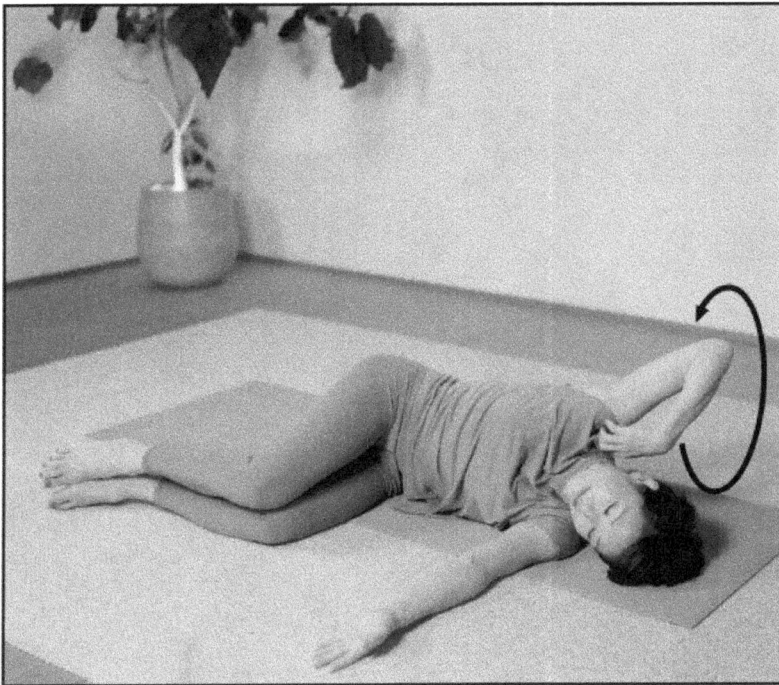

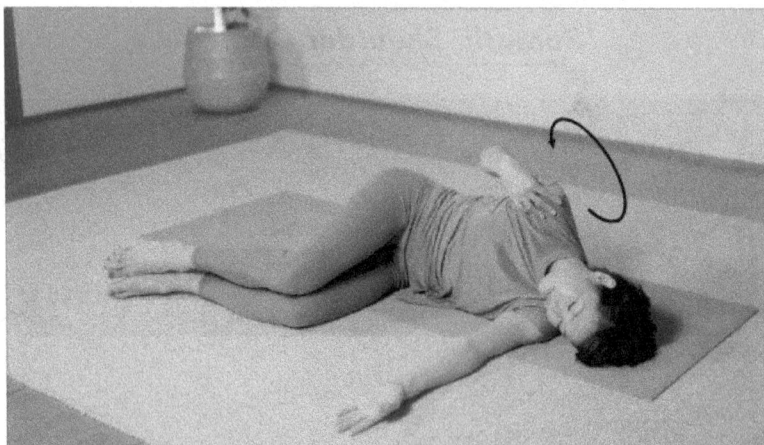

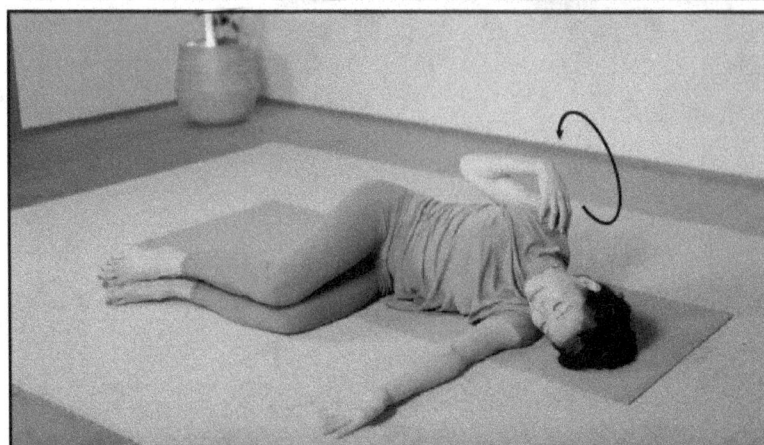

- Slowly move your elbow in a gentle circle, noticing your shoulder blade sliding.

- Inhale as the elbow lifts, exhale as it softens down.

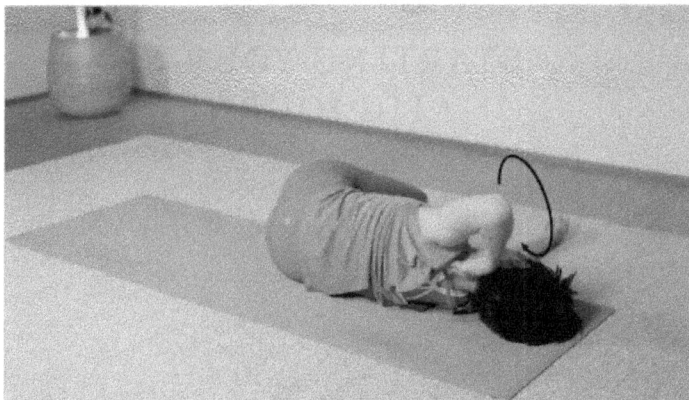

- After 4–6 circles, reverse the direction.

- Pause and rest your arm by your side.

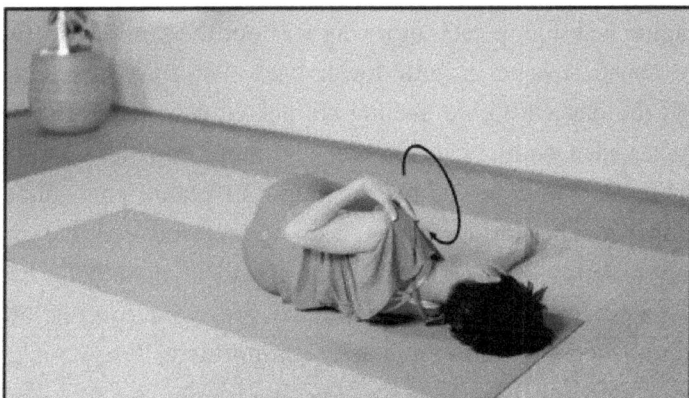

- Notice the difference in sensation between the worked side and the resting side.

- Repeat with the opposite hand and shoulder.

CHAPTER 2

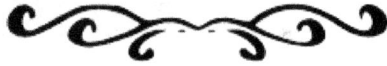

STARTING YOUR SOMATIC JOURNEY

Imagine waking up each morning without the familiar stiffness or the constant ache in your lower back. Picture yourself moving through the day with ease, feeling connected to your body in a way that makes each moment feel lighter and more effortless. This vision isn't far-fetched or reserved for the few; it's a reality you can achieve with Somatic Therapy Exercises. Many people believe that starting any new practice requires a drastic overhaul of their daily life. But Somatic Therapy Exercises fit seamlessly into your routine, offering profound benefits with minimal daily commitment.

To begin, it's crucial to establish a routine that feels manageable. Consistency, not intensity, is your guiding principle here. Rather than aiming for long, strenuous sessions, focus on short, regular practices you can easily maintain. A good starting point might be dedicating ten to fifteen minutes each morning to your practice. This time can be your moment of calm before the day unfolds. Alternatively, you might find evenings more suitable, using the exercises to wind down and release the day's tensions.

A simple daily schedule could look like this: begin with a basic body scan. This exercise helps you tune into your body, identifying areas of tension or discomfort. Take a few moments to close your eyes, breathe deeply, and mentally scan from the top of your head to the tips of your toes. Notice any sensations without judgment. This practice helps build awareness and sets the tone for the exercises to follow. Next, incorporate introductory breathing techniques, such as deep diaphragmatic breathing. Place one hand on your chest and the other on your belly. Breathe in slowly through your nose, allowing your belly to rise. Exhale gently, allowing your abdomen to relax and fall. This technique calms the nervous system and prepares your body for movement.

As you become more comfortable, add a weekly routine with more varied exercises. On weekends, you can extend your practice to include gentle stretching or movements that target specific areas, such as the neck or shoulders. These sessions can last twenty to thirty minutes, providing a more comprehensive reset for the week ahead.

Staying motivated can sometimes be a challenge. It's easy to start with enthusiasm, only to have it wane over time. Keeping a practice log or journal can help maintain your commitment. Use it to note how you feel before and after each session, or jot down any changes you notice. This simple reflection can highlight progress and reinforce the benefits you're experiencing.

Additionally, consider joining an online somatic community. Sharing your journey with others can offer support and encouragement. You might exchange tips, celebrate milestones, or connect with others who understand the challenges and triumphs of incorporating Somatic Therapy Exercises into daily life.

Remember, the goal isn't perfection but rather a steady, gentle progression toward greater awareness and ease. By setting realistic goals for your practice frequency, you avoid the pitfalls of overexertion and burnout. If you miss a day or two, don't be discouraged. Return to your practice with kindness and patience, knowing that each session contributes to your overall well-being.

Somatic Therapy Exercises provide an opportunity to reconnect with yourself in a meaningful way. They invite you to explore your body's potential, not through force or discipline but through awareness and understanding. As you build your routine, celebrate the small victories and remain open to the insights gained from each practice. With time and consistency, you'll find that these exercises transform how you move, feel, and engage with the world around you.

2.1 ESSENTIAL TOOLS AND PROPS FOR EFFECTIVE PRACTICE

Getting started with Somatic Therapy Exercises doesn't require a lot of equipment. Still, a few key tools can enhance your practice and make it more comfortable. A yoga mat is a great place to start. It provides a cushioned surface for floor exercises, protecting your joints and offering a stable base. Choose a mat that suits your needs. Some prefer a thicker mat for extra cushioning, which can be helpful if you have sensitive knees or a back. Others might opt for a thinner mat for better balance. You can find mats in various materials and textures, so consider what feels best for you. If you're practicing at home, have enough space to stretch out fully on your mat without bumping into furniture.

Foam rollers are another helpful tool. They help release muscle tension and improve flexibility. You can use a foam roller to gently massage tight areas, such as your back or legs, breaking up knots and enhancing blood flow. When selecting a foam roller, consider its density. Softer rollers provide a gentler massage, which might be more comfortable if you're new to this type of release. Firmer rollers provide deeper pressure, which can be beneficial for targeting stubborn areas. Start with a softer option if unsure, and gradually work to a firmer roller as your body adapts.

Props aren't just about comfort—they can also help you maintain proper posture during exercises. For instance, if you struggle with balance, a yoga block can support your poses, allowing you to focus on alignment without straining. The block can extend your reach, helping you maintain posture without overextending your body. This support is crucial, especially as you begin to explore new movements.

While specialized equipment can be beneficial, you can also get creative with items you have at home. Towels can serve as makeshift yoga straps, helping you hold stretches and improve flexibility. Roll or fold them to the desired thickness and use them to extend your reach during stretches. Cushions or pillows can provide extra support during seated exercises. Place them under your knees or lower back to ease pressure and maintain comfort. These everyday items can significantly impact your practice, ensuring you stay comfortable and supported.

When choosing tools, consider your comfort levels. What feels good for you? What helps you relax and focus? It's important to select items that enhance your experience rather than distract you. The right props can make your practice more enjoyable and effective, allowing you to concentrate on the exercises and the sensations they bring.

Check Your Comfort

- Do you have a yoga mat that feels right for your body?
- Have you tried using a foam roller? How does it feel on your muscles?
- Look around your home: can you find a towel or cushion to support your practice?

Integrating these tools creates a supportive environment for your Somatic Therapy Exercises. They help you connect with your body, letting you explore movements with ease and awareness. Each session becomes a space for discovery, where you can listen to your body's cues and respond to its needs. This mindful approach enriches your practice and fosters a deeper connection with yourself. As you experiment with different tools and props, you'll find what works best for you, enhancing comfort and focus.

2.2 INTEGRATING SOMATIC THERAPY EXERCISES INTO A BUSY LIFESTYLE

Finding time for Somatic Therapy Exercises in a busy schedule can seem daunting. Still, small changes can make a big difference. The key is to identify little pockets of time throughout your day. Imagine your routine like a jar filled with large rocks representing your most significant tasks. The remaining space for small pebbles, such as Somatic Therapy Exercises, can be filled around them efficiently. Look for gaps between tasks. Ten minutes may be before breakfast or a short pause before a meeting. These moments can become opportunities for quick, practical sessions. Prioritizing shorter practices over longer ones ensures consistency without feeling overwhelmed.

Flexibility in your routine is crucial. Life can be unpredictable, with schedules that change unexpectedly. You might plan a morning session, but something comes up. Instead of skipping it entirely, adjust your practice time. You could fit it into your lunch break or before bed. Being adaptable means you can maintain your practice even when life gets busy. This approach keeps you engaged without adding stress. Consider the ebb and flow of your day and be open to shifting your practice as needed.

Quick exercises are perfect for busy days. Desk stretches offer a simple way to release tension without leaving your chair. Try rolling your shoulders back and down or gently twisting from side to side to ease stiffness. For a mental reset, a five-minute breathing exercise can work wonders. Sit comfortably, close your eyes, and take a deep breath. Focus on each inhale and exhale, letting the rhythm calm your mind. These exercises are easy to incorporate into any schedule, providing quick relief and helping you feel centered.

Staying focused amidst distractions can be challenging. Creating a dedicated practice space can help. Select a quiet corner in your home or office where you feel at ease. This space becomes your sanctuary, where you can focus solely on your practice. It doesn't need to be large, just a spot where you can stretch and breathe without interruption. Setting reminders or alarms for practice time also keeps you on track. A gentle nudge on your phone can prompt you to pause and engage with your exercises, even on the busiest days.

With these strategies, Somatic Therapy Exercises can become a natural part of your day. They don't require hours of commitment, just a mindful approach and the willingness to seize moments that might otherwise go unnoticed. By integrating exercises into your routine, you create a rhythm that supports your well-being, even when life feels hectic. This consistency can lead to profound benefits, allowing you to navigate daily challenges with greater ease and resilience. The more you practice, the more you'll notice positive changes in how you feel and move.

2.3 ADDRESSING BEGINNER CONCERNS: FLEXIBILITY AND TIME CONSTRAINTS

Starting something new can be daunting, especially when it feels like flexibility is a distant goal. But Somatic Therapy Exercises cater to all levels of flexibility, welcoming everyone into the practice with open arms. They are not about forcing your body into uncomfortable positions or comparing yourself to others. Instead, they are about working with what you have and celebrating gradual improvements. Modified poses ensure those with limited flexibility can still engage fully. For example, if a full stretch feels out of reach, you can adjust your posture to suit your body by using props or altering the angle. This adaptability is key. It allows you to progress at your own pace, fostering confidence and comfort as you grow stronger and more flexible.

Time often feels like a scarce resource. Many of us struggle to find extra minutes in our packed schedules. That's why time-efficient routines can make all the difference. Imagine a ten-minute routine that fits snugly into a busy morning. It might include a gentle wake-up stretch, a few mindful breaths, and a calming focus exercise. When practiced consistently, these short sessions build up to significant change over time. The power of these brief moments lies in their cumulative effect. A few minutes each day can set the tone for how you feel. They become a buffer against stress, a moment to reset and center yourself before diving into daily demands.

You don't need long, intense workouts to see benefits. Even brief periods of practice can lead to significant improvements. These short sessions are sufficient to notice changes in their movement and overall well-being. One might share how ten minutes each day helped alleviate chronic back pain. Another might mention how morning exercises improved their mood and energy levels. Each story highlights the transformative potential of small, consistent efforts. These examples remind us that every bit counts; even the most minor step forward is progress.

As you begin this practice, remember to be kind to yourself. Patience and self-compassion are your allies. It's easy to feel disheartened if progress seems slow at first. But every expert was once a beginner. Embrace the learning process with grace. Celebrate small victories, like touching your toes or finding peace in a busy day. These achievements serve as stepping stones on your path to improved well-being. Many beginners have faced similar challenges, yet they've persevered and thrived. Their stories of overcoming initial hurdles can inspire you to stay committed, even when the going gets tough. They demonstrate that persistence pays off, and your efforts will yield results over time.

The practice of Somatic Therapy Exercises is more than just physical. It's an invitation to explore and understand your body in a new and different way. It encourages you to listen to your rhythms, to honor your limits, and to find joy in the simple act of moving mindfully. Through this practice, you create a space for self-care and healing. You learn to appreciate your body's capabilities without judgment or pressure. This approach lays a foundation for lasting change, helping you feel more comfortable in your own skin. With each session, you strengthen your connection to your body, enhancing both your physical health and emotional resilience.

2.4 QUICK STRESS RELIEF TECHNIQUES FOR THE WORKPLACE

Stress can sneak up on you in the hustle and bustle of the workday. It tightens your shoulders, clouds your mind, and drains you. But even at your desk, you can find moments of calm. Seated breathing exercises are a simple yet effective way to ease stress. Sit back in your chair, place your feet flat on the ground, and close your eyes if possible. Inhale slowly through your nose, letting your belly expand. Hold for a second, then exhale gently. Repeat this cycle a few times. You'll notice your heart rate slowing, your mind clearing, and your body relaxing.

Neck and shoulder stretches can also provide relief. To start, sit up straight and drop your shoulders away from your ears. Gently tilt your head to one side, allowing the stretch to feel along the opposite side of your neck. Hold for a few breaths, then switch to the other side. Roll your shoulders forward and backward to release tension. These stretches require no special equipment and can be done in minutes. They're perfect for breaking the cycle of stress that often builds up during long hours at the computer.

Short breaks are not just a luxury but are necessary for maintaining focus and productivity. Research suggests that taking regular breaks can improve concentration and reduce fatigue. You might think stepping away for a few minutes could disrupt your workflow, but the opposite is true. A brief pause lets your mind reset, making you more effective upon return. Use these breaks to incorporate somatic exercises. They rejuvenate your body and mind, preparing you to tackle the following task with renewed energy.

In an office setting, specific exercises can target challenges you face daily. For instance, wrist stretches can help prevent stiffness and pain, especially if you spend hours typing. Extend one arm out, palm facing down. Use your other hand to gently pull back on your fingers, feeling the stretch along your forearm. Hold briefly, then switch sides. During stressful meetings, grounding techniques can help you stay centered. Press your feet firmly into the floor, feeling the support beneath you. Focus on this sensation to bring awareness to the present moment, easing anxiety and promoting calm.

Creating a supportive work environment can enhance these practices. Encourage colleagues to join you in group stretching sessions. Propose a five-minute break during team meetings. This fosters camaraderie and emphasizes the importance of stress management at work. Setting up a quiet corner in the office for relaxation exercises can also be beneficial. A small space with a mat or cushion invites you to pause and practice. It signals to others that taking time to de-stress is valued and supported.

As you incorporate these quick stress relief techniques into your daily work routine, you'll find that they fit in seamlessly. They become tools you can rely on, no matter how busy or chaotic your schedule. Regular practice cultivates a sense of calm and control, enabling you to face each challenge with confidence. These exercises are not just about managing stress; they are about enhancing your quality of life. They remind you to listen to your body and prioritize well-being, even in a work environment that often demands the opposite.

With these practices in place, you're ready to explore the world of Somatic Therapy Exercises. The next chapter will delve into how deepening your body awareness can further enhance your physical and emotional well-being.

Diaphragmatic Breathing with Hands on Belly

○ Sit or lie down comfortably. Place one hand on your chest and one on your belly.

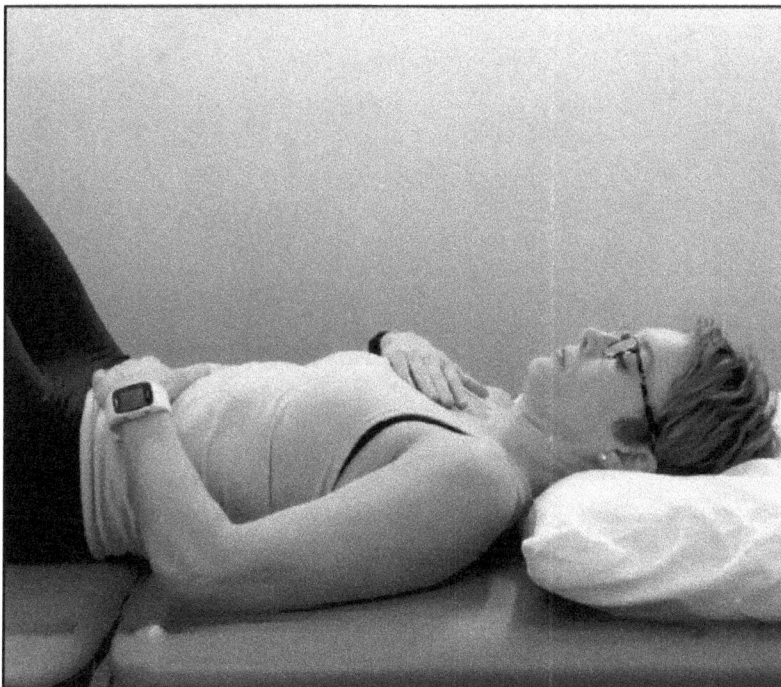

Inhale slowly through your nose, letting your belly rise while your chest stays mostly still.

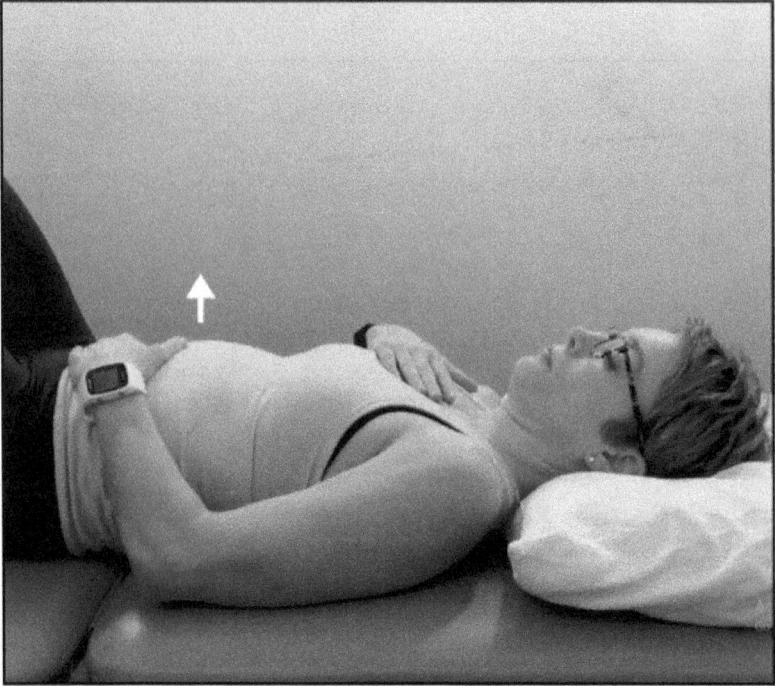

- Exhale gently through your mouth.

- Feel your belly fall as you release the air, maintaining a smooth, steady flow.

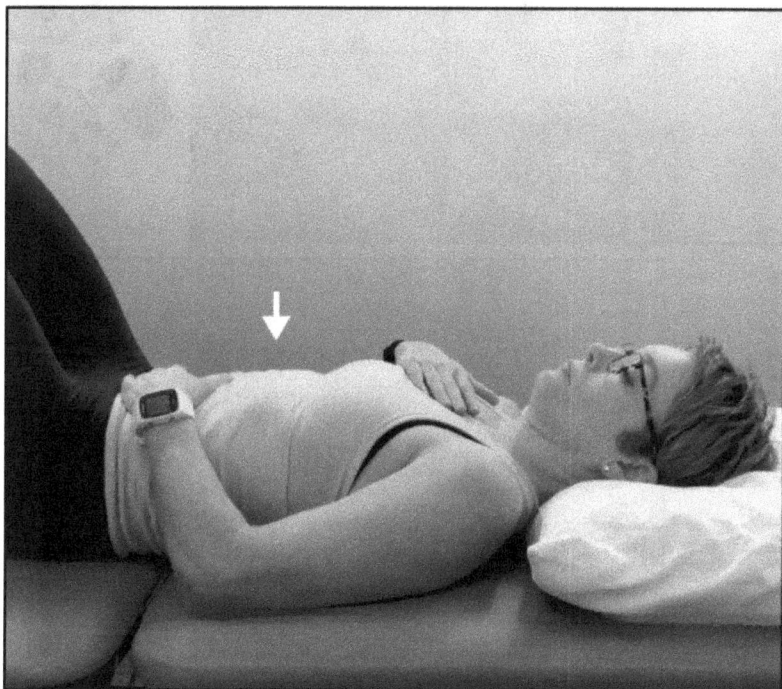

- Continue for 5-10 slow breaths.

- Maintain awareness of your hand movements—belly rising on inhale, belly falling on exhale.

Wrist and Forearm Stretch

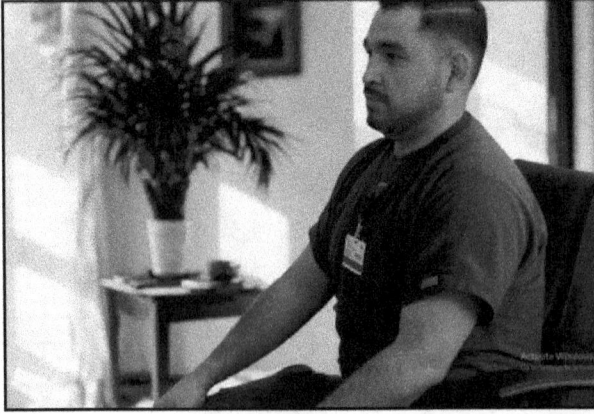

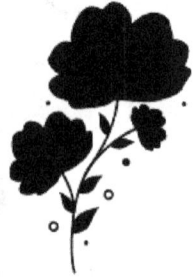

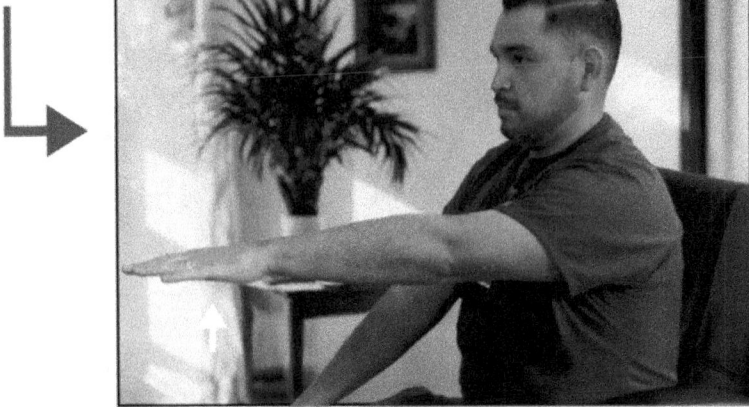

- Sit or stand with your spine upright and shoulders relaxed.

- Extend your left arm straight out in front of you at shoulder height, palm facing down.

38

- With your right hand, gently pull down on your extended hand, guiding them downward until you feel a stretch along the underside of your forearm.

- Keep your elbow straight but not locked.

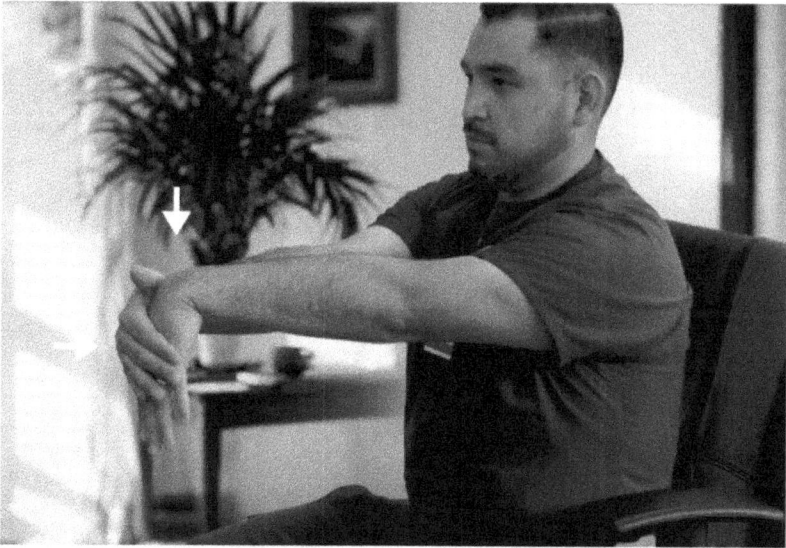

- Turn your left palm up.

- Use your right hand to press the palm of your left hand, guiding your fingers toward your body to stretch the top of your forearm.

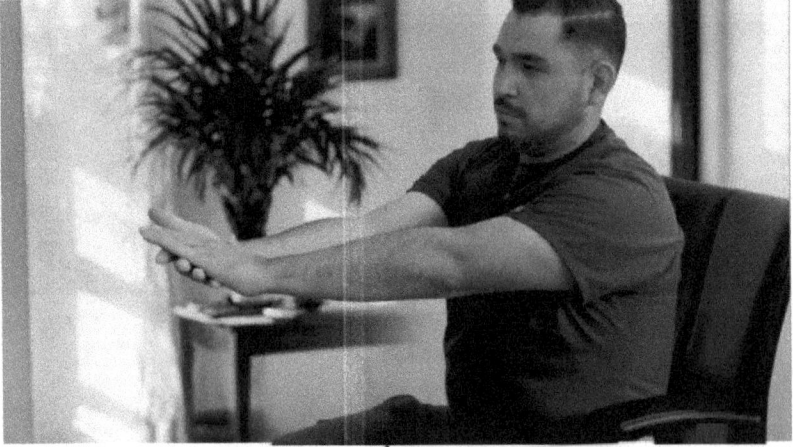

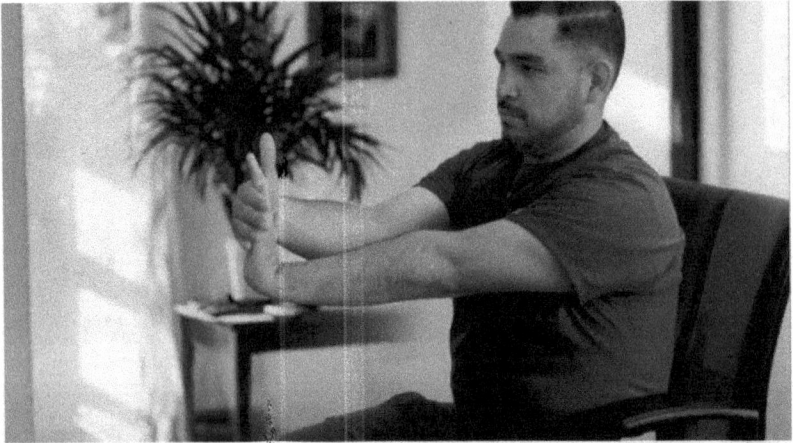

- Hold each stretch for 10–15 seconds.

- Switch arms and repeat the same procedure 2–3 times per side.

CHAPTER 3

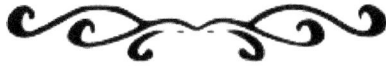

DEEPENING BODY AWARENESS AND EMOTIONAL CONNECTION

I magine standing at the edge of a serene lake, its surface smooth and undisturbed. Toss a pebble into this lake and watch the ripples spread, touching every corner. This image captures the essence of a body scan. Much like how ripples move across water, a body scan allows awareness to flow through you, reaching every part. This practice is rooted in mindfulness, an ancient tradition that teaches us to observe without judgment. Historically, it has been used to cultivate a deeper understanding of the body and mind, drawing from teachings in Buddhist meditation practices (Source 1). This simple act can reconnect you with yourself in today's fast-paced world, offering clarity and peace.

To begin a body scan, find a quiet, comfortable place. Lie down or sit in a chair with both feet on the floor. Close your eyes if you feel comfortable, and take a few deep breaths. Start by focusing on your toes. Notice any sensations, whether warmth, coolness, or even tingling. Then, slowly move your attention up to your feet, ankles, and calves. Continue this journey through your body, moving to your knees, thighs, and hips. Take a moment to connect with each part, acknowledging any tension or comfort you may feel. As you reach your torso, notice how your chest rises and falls with each breath. Feel your shoulders, arms, and fingers, then move up to your neck and face. End at the top of your head, taking a deep breath to conclude the scan. If your mind wanders during this process, gently bring it back to the body part you're focusing on. This practice trains your mind to stay present, fostering patience and concentration.

The benefits of regular body scans are numerous. They can significantly reduce stress and anxiety levels. By becoming more aware of your body, you learn to release tension before it builds. This practice can also improve sleep quality. As you become attuned to your body, falling asleep becomes more manageable, and rest is more restorative.

Additionally, body scans promote relaxation. They help you unwind and disconnect from daily stressors, creating a sense of calm. This practice benefits your mind and physical health. Regular scans can lower blood pressure and improve circulation, contributing to overall well-being.

Many individuals have experienced these benefits firsthand. Consider Sarah, a teacher who felt overwhelmed by her hectic schedule. After incorporating body scans into her daily routine, she noticed a significant decrease in her anxiety levels. She found she was more present with her students and patient in challenging situations. Another person, Mark, struggled with insomnia for years. Through consistent practice of body scans, he found that his sleep improved dramatically. He fell asleep more quickly and woke up feeling refreshed. These stories highlight the transformative potential of body scans. They help you become more mindful and in tune with your body, leading to positive changes in your life.

Emotion-in-Motion Dance

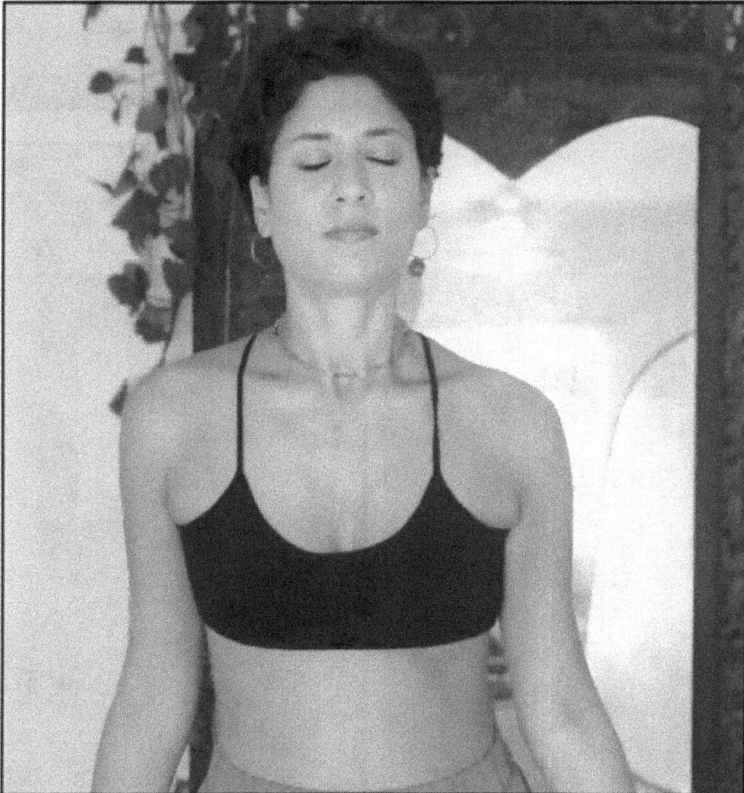

- Stand tall and close your eyes for a moment.

- Notice what you're feeling, without needing to label it perfectly.

- Start moving freely.

- Sway, shake, stretch, or shift your weight — let   the emotion move through your body.

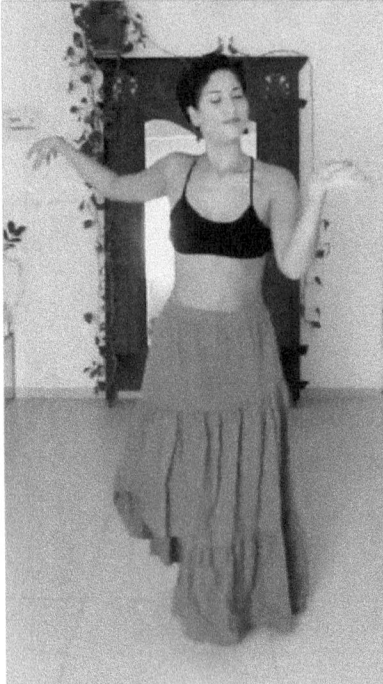

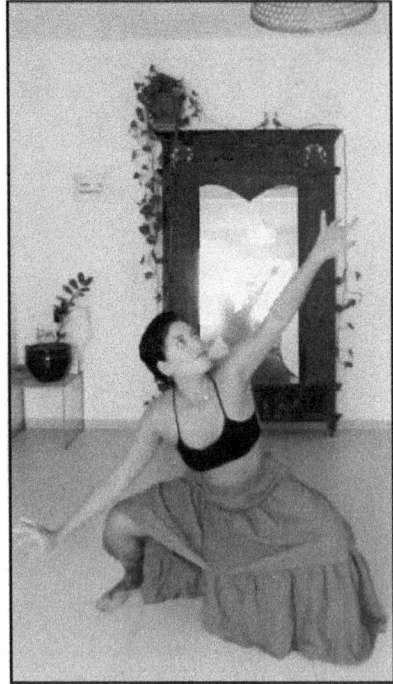

- Keep breathing as you move.

- Let your movement be expressive, not perfect. Fast or slow — follow your feeling.

Slowly return to stillness.

Bring your hands to your heart. Take a deep breath and notice how you feel now.

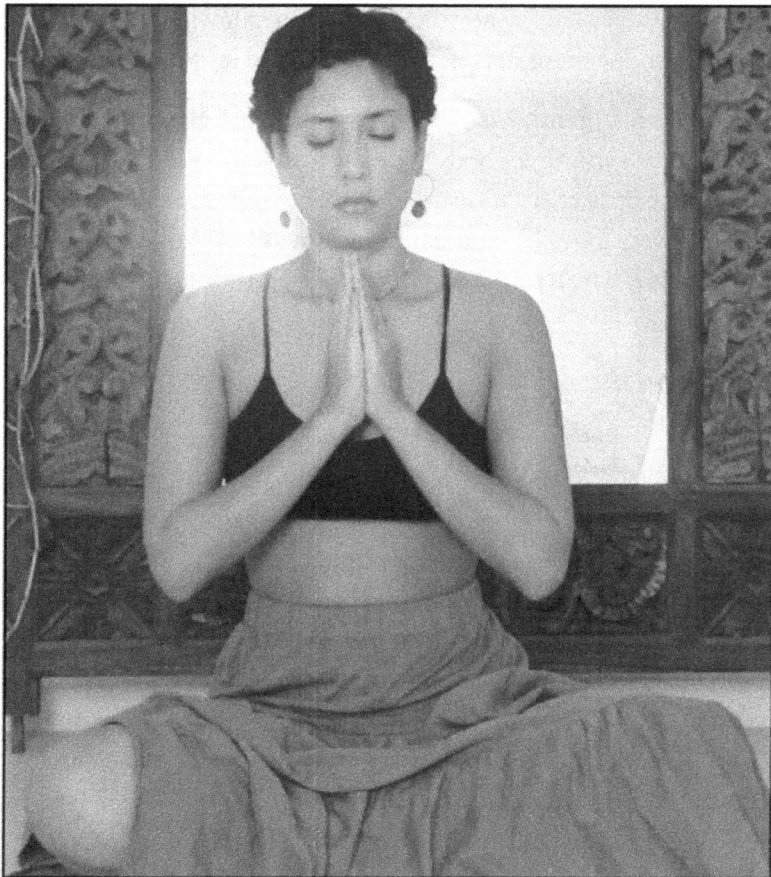

Interactive Exercise: Your Body Scan Journal

Start a journal to document your body scan experiences. After each session, write down your observations. Note any areas of tension or comfort, as well as how you felt before and after the scan. Over time, look for patterns or changes that emerge. Reflect on how this practice influences your mood, stress levels, and overall well-being. This exercise encourages self-awareness and helps you track your progress. It also provides a space for personal reflection, allowing you to explore the deeper connections between your body and mind.

Body scans are potent tools for self-discovery and healing. They invite you to explore your own body with curiosity and kindness. Through this practice, you can cultivate a deeper connection with yourself, enhancing your physical and emotional health. As you continue with these exercises, you'll find they bring peace and clarity to your life.

3.1 EXPLORING EMOTIONAL LANDSCAPES THROUGH MOVEMENT

Emotions and movement are closely linked, like the wind and the branches it stirs. When you feel something deeply, it often shows in how you move. Notice how anger might cause your fists to clench or how joy can make you leap. Emotions are not just thoughts in your head. They live in your body, too. Moving your body can help release emotions, allowing them to flow out instead of staying stuck inside. Movement can help process what words sometimes cannot express. This is because physical activity can touch parts of your emotional experience that remain out of reach with thoughts alone. When you move, you tangibly engage with your emotions.

To explore your emotions through movement, begin with simple exercises. Dance-like movements can be very freeing. Put on music that speaks to you and let your body move however it wants. It doesn't have to look a certain way. The goal is to feel, not perform. Let your arms swing, your feet tap, or your head sway. This movement can help release emotions that are stuck inside, such as stress or sadness. Another approach is to move slowly and deliberately. Try standing with your feet shoulder-width apart. Gently sway from side to side, feeling the weight shift from one foot to the other. Notice how each movement feels. This can help you tune into emotions you may not be aware of carrying.

Movement as a tool for healing has a long history. Many people have found comfort and understanding through movement-based therapy. For example, dance therapy is used to help people process trauma and express difficult-to-speak-of feelings. One case study tells of a woman who, through therapeutic dance, worked through the grief she had held for years. She found new ways to express and release her emotions in each session. Stories like hers show how movement can lead to personal transformation.

Another example is a man who used movement to cope with anxiety. By practicing daily movements, he discovered a sense of calm and control. This highlights the therapeutic potential of moving with intention.

To deepen your emotional exploration, try keeping a movement journal. After each session, take a moment to jot down what you felt. You might note which movements felt good and which emotions surfaced. Reflect on any changes you notice in yourself. This practice can help you track your progress and gain valuable insights over time. Consider prompts like, "What emotions did I notice during my movement?" or "How did my body feel before and after?" Documenting your experiences can reveal patterns and growth, offering a clearer picture of your emotional landscape. This reflection can also remind you of the healing power you've found in movement.

Movement is not just about exercise; it's a way to connect with yourself on a deeper, more profound level. It invites you to explore and express emotions that might otherwise remain hidden. Engaging in these practices opens the door to understanding and healing. As you move, you listen to your body and emotions, gaining a deeper understanding of your inner world. This connection can bring about significant change, helping you feel more grounded and connected to yourself. Through movement, you find a language that speaks directly to your emotions, offering a path toward healing and self-discovery.

3.2 TECHNIQUES FOR ENHANCING MINDFUL MOVEMENT

Imagine walking through a park, feeling the ground beneath your feet and the breeze brushing against your skin. This scenario captures the essence of mindful movement, which involves being fully present while engaging in physical activity. It's about focusing on every step and every breath, allowing you to connect deeply with your body. The mindful movement combines physical activity with mindfulness, a practice of being aware of the moment without judgment. This method can significantly boost your focus and concentration. When you engage in mindful movement, your mind learns to quiet down, letting you concentrate on the task at hand. This focus not only benefits you during exercises, but also in other areas of your life. It spills over into your daily life, allowing you to handle tasks more clearly and with less stress.

The mindful movement also enhances the synchronization between your body and mind. When your actions and thoughts align, you experience a sense of balance and calm. This connection fosters a deeper understanding of how your body responds to stress or relaxation. You become more aware of your physical and emotional states, which allows you to make more informed choices about your well-being. This practice can enhance mental health, alleviate anxiety, and foster a more profound sense of peace. By integrating mindfulness with movement, you cultivate a holistic approach to health that addresses both physical and emotional needs.

Let's explore some exercises that highlight this integration. Walking meditation is a great place to start. As you walk, focus on the sensations in your feet. Notice how they lift and touch the ground. Feel the muscles in your legs and the rhythm of your breath. Walking meditation is not about reaching a destination. It's about the journey itself and being present with each step. Another exercise involves yoga-inspired mindful stretching. Begin with a simple pose, like a forward bend. As you stretch, pay attention to your breath and the sensations in your muscles. Hold the position for a few breaths, noticing how your body feels. These exercises encourage your presence and engagement, fostering a deeper connection with your body.

Setting intentions plays a crucial role in mindful movement. Before you begin, take a moment to set a clear intention for your practice. This intention could be as simple as focusing on your breath or being kind to yourself. Setting intentions gives your practice a purpose, guiding your actions and thoughts. It transforms your movement from a routine activity into a meaningful one. Intentions also influence the quality of your movement. When you move with intention, you become more mindful of each action, which can lead to more effective and satisfying experiences. This awareness helps you stay engaged and connected to your practice, enhancing its benefits.

Incorporating breathwork into mindful movement can further enhance the practice. Breath serves as a powerful anchor, keeping you grounded and focused. Synchronizing your breath with movement can deepen your awareness and improve the quality of your exercise. For example, try inhaling as you lift your arms and exhaling as you lower them. This simple technique encourages a smooth flow of movement, promoting relaxation and reducing tension. Controlled breathing also benefits your overall well-being. It helps regulate your nervous system, lowers stress, and increases oxygen flow to your brain. These benefits contribute to a more balanced and centered state of being during and after your practice.

Mindful movement offers a path to greater awareness and well-being. Integrating mindfulness, intention, and breath into your exercises creates a practice that nurtures both body and mind. This approach encourages you to listen to your body's cues, fostering a deeper connection with yourself. Through mindful movement, you can discover a sense of peace and balance that enhances all aspects of your life.

3.3 BUILDING EMOTIONAL RESILIENCE WITH SOMATIC PRACTICES

Emotional resilience is the ability to bounce back from stress and challenges. It's like a muscle that strengthens with use. When you build resilience, you become more adaptable to life's ups and downs. It helps you manage stress more effectively so you're not overwhelmed by every little setback. Emotionally resilient individuals tend to remain calm in challenging situations. They view challenges as opportunities for growth rather than threats. This mindset not only helps with stress management; it also enhances overall well-being. It also boosts mental health, making you more confident and less prone to anxiety or depression.

Somatic practices, which focus on body awareness, can be a powerful way to build this resilience. One simple exercise is grounding. Imagine you're a tree with roots extending deep into the earth. Stand or sit comfortably and feel the ground beneath you. This exercise can stabilize your emotions, helping you feel more secure and less anxious. Another technique is focused breathing. When stress strikes, take a few deep breaths to calm yourself. Inhale slowly, hold for a moment, then exhale gently. This helps regulate emotions and brings a sense of calm. Both exercises are easy to practice at any time and in any place. They allow you to stay connected to the present moment, reducing the impact of stress.

Practicing somatic exercises regularly can lead to significant improvements in emotional health. Over time, you'll notice that your ability to handle stress improves. You might find yourself less reactive and more thoughtful in challenging situations. This change doesn't happen overnight, but it becomes a natural part of your life with consistency and persistence. The benefits of building emotional resilience are long-lasting. They extend to many areas of your life, from relationships to work. When you're resilient, you're better equipped to face life's challenges with confidence and grace. This emotional strength can also protect you from the effects of chronic stress, promoting overall well-being.

Real-life stories demonstrate the transformative power of somatic practices in fostering resilience. Take Jenny, for example. She struggled with anxiety for years, often feeling overwhelmed by daily tasks. After incorporating grounding exercises into her routine, she noticed a shift. She felt more centered and less anxious. Another story is about Tom, who used focused breathing to manage his stress at work. It helped him stay calm during essential meetings, improving his performance and confidence. These examples highlight how somatic practices can enhance coping skills and adaptability.

Many people find that these practices enhance their emotional resilience, leading to personal growth and transformation. As you become more attuned to your body and emotions, you see yourself in a new light. You discover strengths you didn't know you had, empowering you to tackle challenges with a more positive approach. This newfound confidence can open doors to new opportunities, both personally and professionally.

Incorporating somatic practices into your life can be a simple yet powerful way to enhance emotional resilience. The exercises are easy to learn and can be done anywhere, making them accessible to everyone. As you practice, you build a foundation of strength and stability that supports you through life's ups and downs. This resilience is about enduring stress and thriving despite it, turning obstacles into stepping stones for growth.

Side-to-Side Weight Shift (Sway Practice)

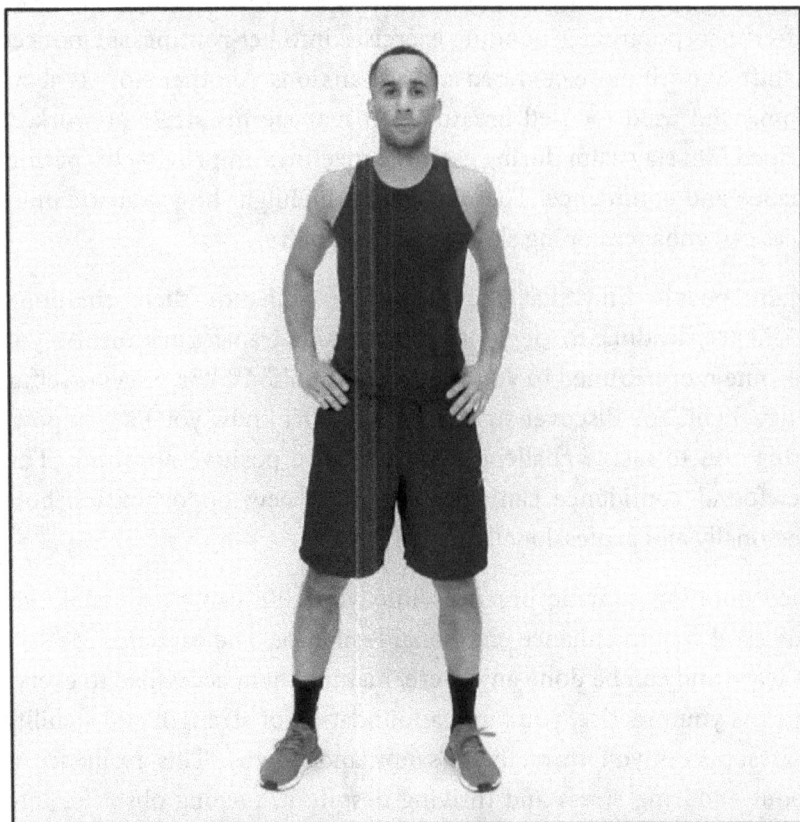

○ Stand with your feet hip-width apart and your knees slightly bent.

○ Let your arms hang naturally by your sides or place your hands on your hips.

○ Relax your shoulders and keep your gaze soft or gently forward.

- Slowly shift your body weight to your right foot.

- Allow your hips to move slightly to the right and your left heel to lift lightly off the ground.

- Then shift your weight to the left side, letting your right heel lift in return.

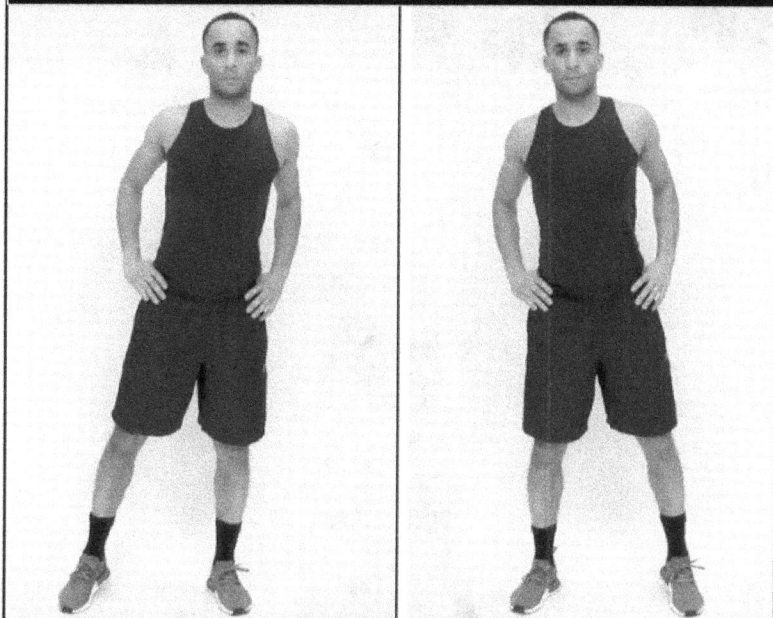

- Inhale as you shift to one side, exhale as you sway to the other.

- Move rhythmically, keeping the knees soft and the motion smooth.

- Let the movement be natural and unforced, like gentle rocking.

- Continue swaying side to side for 8–10 slow cycles.

- Stay connected to your feet, breath, and center of gravity.

- To finish, return to center and stand still for a few breaths to absorb the effects.

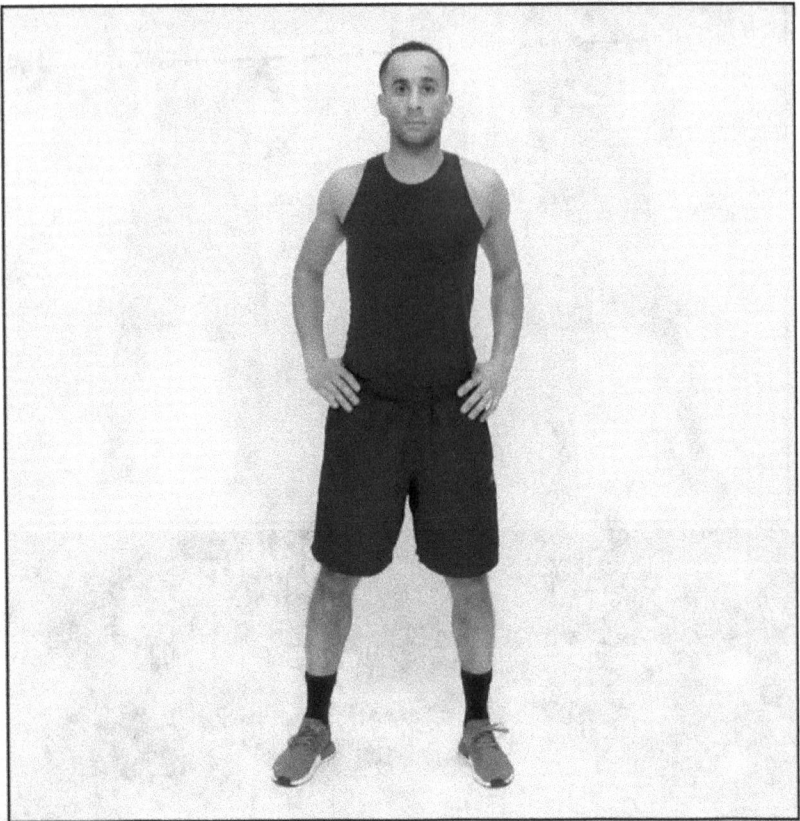

3.4 THE POWER OF VISUALIZATION IN SOMATIC EXERCISES

Visualization is a powerful tool that can enhance your practice of somatic exercises. It involves creating mental images that can help guide your physical actions. When you visualize, you engage parts of your brain that are actually in motion. This mental rehearsal can strengthen the connection between your mind and body. Visualization taps into cognitive processes that help you learn and remember new skills. It can be as effective as physical practice because your brain interprets imagined actions as if they were real ones. Athletes often use visualization to prepare for competitions. They mentally run through their routines, which helps improve their performance. In somatic exercises, visualization aids in releasing tension and promoting relaxation. By imagining specific outcomes, you can enhance your physical and emotional awareness.

To practice visualization, find a quiet place where you can sit or lie down comfortably. Close your eyes and take a few deep breaths. Begin by imagining a place that makes you feel calm and peaceful. It could be a beach, a forest, or anywhere you feel relaxed. Picture the details, like the sounds you hear or the colors you see. Now, focus on an area of your body that feels tense. Visualize warmth and light flowing into that area, melting away any tension. Imagine your muscles softening and relaxing. Continue this process, moving your attention through different parts of your body. Use your imagination to create a sense of peace and ease. This exercise can help you become more aware of how your body holds stress and how to release it.

There are many benefits to combining visualization with somatic practices. It can enhance your focus and concentration. When you visualize, you train your mind to stay present and engaged. This focus enables you to perform exercises with greater precision and effectiveness. Visualization also improves emotional processing and regulation. By imagining positive outcomes, you can shift your mindset and reduce stress. This technique enables you to explore emotions safely, facilitating a deeper understanding and practical working through of them. Visualization enhances your somatic practice, creating a richer and more fulfilling experience.

Many people have found success using visualization in their somatic exercises. Take Jane, for example. She struggled with chronic tension in her shoulders. Through visualization, she learned to imagine her shoulders softening and relaxing. Over time, this practice helped her reduce pain and increase mobility. Another person, Tom, used visualization to enhance his focus during meditation. He imagined a beam of light connecting his mind and body. This image helped him stay grounded and present, leading to greater clarity and peace. These stories show how visualization can transform your practice and help you achieve your goals.

Visualization is more than just a mental exercise. It's a way to connect your mind and body, enhancing your overall well-being. By incorporating visualization into your somatic practice, you can unlock new levels of awareness and healing. This technique encourages you to explore and use your imagination to support your physical and emotional health. As you continue to practice, you'll discover the power of your mind to influence your body and create positive change. Visualization enriches your experience, providing a powerful tool for growth and transformation.

This chapter explored different ways to deepen your connection to your body and emotions. We looked at body scans, mindful movement, and visualization. These practices invite you to listen to your body and understand your feelings. They build a foundation for healing and growth. The next chapter will address stress, anxiety, and tension. These are common challenges that somatic exercises can help manage. Integrating these practices into your life can enhance your well-being and help you navigate life's challenges more easily.

CHAPTER 4

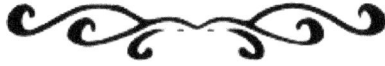

ADDRESSING STRESS, ANXIETY, AND TENSION

S tress often feels like a constant companion, lurking in the background and waiting to pounce at the slightest hint of pressure. It might be the tightness in your chest before a meeting or the racing thoughts that keep you awake at night. These feelings can weigh heavily on your mind and body, leaving you exhausted and overwhelmed. Yet, there's a tool that can offer relief and calm: breathwork. This simple yet effective technique involves controlled breathing to help manage stress and its physical symptoms. When stress strikes, your body reacts with a "fight or flight" response. Your heart rate increases, your muscles tense, and your mind races. Breathwork helps counteract these effects by engaging your parasympathetic nervous system, which promotes relaxation and recovery. Focusing on your breath can shift your body's response from stress to calm, reducing anxiety and tension.

The parasympathetic nervous system plays a crucial role in stress reduction. It works like a brake, slowing down your body's stress responses and promoting a state of rest. When you practice breathwork, you activate this system, encouraging your body to relax and recover. This process lowers your heart rate, reduces muscle tension, and calms your mind. For example, when you inhale deeply and exhale slowly, your body receives signals to release tension and stress. This practice can help you feel more centered and in control, even in stressful situations.

Several breathwork techniques can help you manage stress. One popular method is box breathing, which involves a simple pattern: inhale for four counts, hold for four counts, exhale for four counts, and hold again for four counts. This technique helps calm the mind and regain focus. Another approach is diaphragmatic breathing, which promotes relaxation by encouraging deep, slow breaths. To practice this, place one hand on your chest and the other on your abdomen. As you inhale, let your abdomen expand, then exhale slowly, feeling your abdomen fall. This method enhances relaxation and reduces stress. Alternate nostril breathing is another technique to help balance and focus your mind. Close your right nostril with your thumb, then inhale through your left nostril. Next, switch your finger to close your left nostril and exhale through your right. Repeat this pattern for several breaths. This exercise can help create a sense of balance and calm.

Consistent breathwork practice offers numerous benefits. It enhances emotional regulation, allowing you to manage stress with greater ease. Practicing these techniques trains your mind and body to respond calmly to stressors. Your concentration and mental clarity also improve, making it easier to focus on tasks and think clearly. The more you practice, the more your body and mind learn to operate in a relaxed state, reducing the impact of stress on your daily life.

Integrating breathwork into your daily routine can be simple. You might set aside time for morning or evening sessions, incorporating breathwork into your self-care routine. Find a quiet, comfortable space where you can practice without interruptions. Whether it's a few minutes in the morning to set the tone for your day or a session before bed to unwind, these practices can help you center and ground yourself. You can also use breathwork during stressful situations. Next time you feel overwhelmed, pause and focus on your breath. This quick reset can help you regain control and calm your mind.

Interactive Element: Your Breathwork Practice Checklist

- **Morning Session**: Spend 5-10 minutes practicing a breathwork technique of your choice. Notice how it sets the tone for your day.
- **During Stress**: When feeling stressed, take a moment to practice box breathing. Observe how it helps you regain focus and calm.
- **Evening Session**: Wind down your day with 5-10 minutes of diaphragmatic breathing. Reflect on how it aids relaxation before sleep.

Breathwork is a powerful tool for managing stress and anxiety. Incorporating these techniques into your life creates a foundation for resilience and well-being. These practices help you navigate life's challenges calmly and confidently, transforming your experience of stress.

4.1 GROUNDING TECHNIQUES FOR ANXIETY RELIEF

Life often feels like a whirlwind. The mind races, bouncing from one worry to the next, leaving you anxious and overwhelmed. In such times, grounding techniques can be your anchor. These methods help you stay present, pulling you away from spiraling thoughts and back into the moment. Grounding works by engaging your senses and refocusing your attention on the physical world. This shift can calm your mind and body, reducing anxiety. The brain benefits from this process as it interrupts the cycle of anxious thoughts. Focusing on the present moment allows your mind to pause and reset.

One grounding technique is the 5-4-3-2-1 sensory method. This exercise uses your senses to bring you back to the present. Start by noticing five things you can see around you. It might be the color of the walls or the shape of a nearby tree. Then, focus on four things you can touch. Feel the texture of your clothing or the smoothness of a table. Next, identify three things you can hear. Listen for the hum of a fan or the sound of birds singing outside. Move on to two things you can smell. It might be your soap or a cup of coffee. Finally, notice one thing you can taste, like toothpaste or gum. This exercise grounds you in reality, easing anxiety and bringing clarity.

Walking barefoot is another grounding method. This simple act connects you directly with the earth, providing stability. As you walk, feel the texture of the ground beneath your feet. Whether grass, sand, or soil, this connection helps root you in the present. Walking barefoot can also reduce stress and improve mood. The natural world has a calming effect, encouraging relaxation and peace. Try this practice in a safe and comfortable space, such as your backyard or a nearby park.

Progressive muscle relaxation is a physical grounding technique that involves tensing and relaxing different muscle groups. Begin with your toes, curling them tightly and then releasing them. Move to your calves, thighs, and other areas, and then to your neck and face. This method releases tension and promotes relaxation. Focusing on each muscle group distracts your mind from anxious thoughts. This practice also helps you become more aware of where you hold tension, allowing you to address it directly.

The benefits of grounding extend beyond the moment. Regular practice can improve your mental health and reduce anxiety symptoms. You may notice fewer panic attacks and less frequent anxious episodes. Grounding techniques help you build resilience, making it easier to cope with stress and anxiety. As you become more adept at these methods, you'll find it easier to remain calm and centered, even in challenging situations.

Consider the story of Lisa, who struggled with daily anxiety. She felt trapped in her thoughts, unable to focus on her work or enjoy time with friends. She learned the 5-4-3-2-1 method and practiced it whenever anxiety struck. Over time, Lisa noticed a change. Her mind felt more apparent, and she could handle stress more efficiently. Similarly, Tom found solace in barefoot walks. He used them as a break from his hectic schedule, allowing him to recharge and return to tasks with renewed energy. These real-life examples show how grounding can transform your experience of anxiety, offering a path to peace and presence.

Evening Relaxation Flow (Legs Up the Wall)

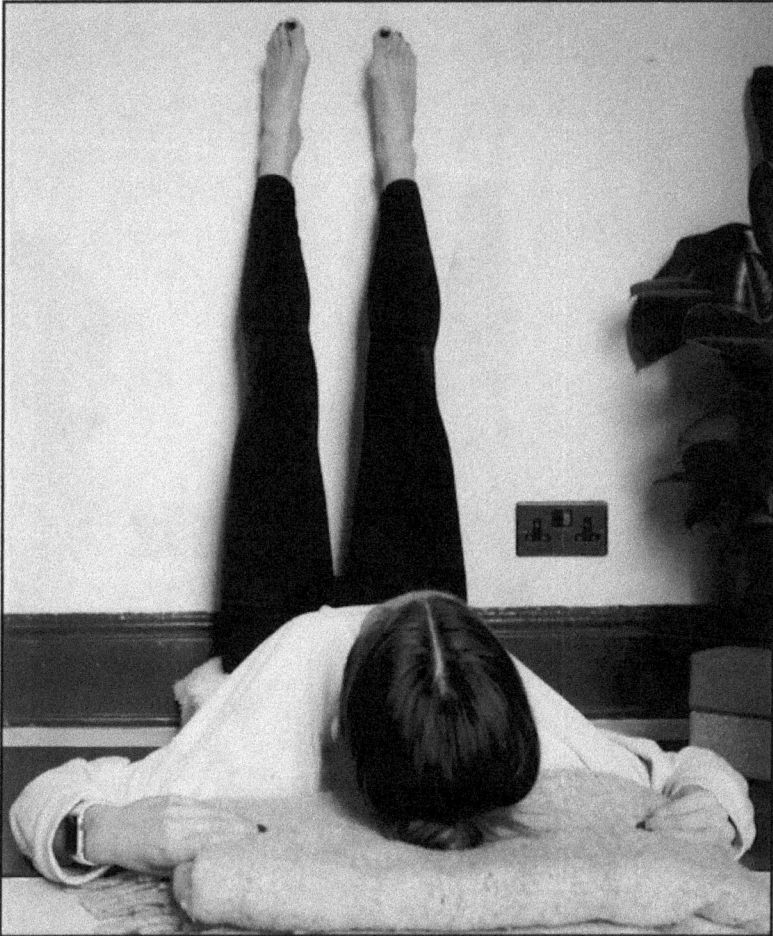

Lie on your back and rest your legs up the wall.

- Place arms by your sides, palms up, and close your eyes.

- Breathe slowly, releasing tension with each exhale.

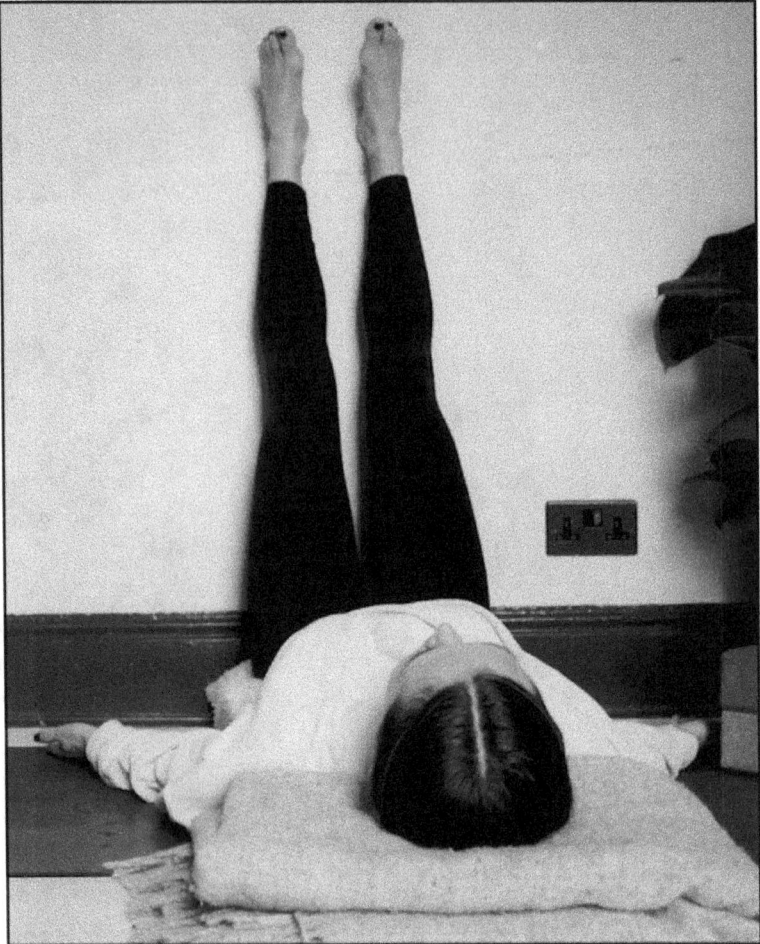

Stay for 3–5 minutes, breathing slowly, then roll to your side to come up.

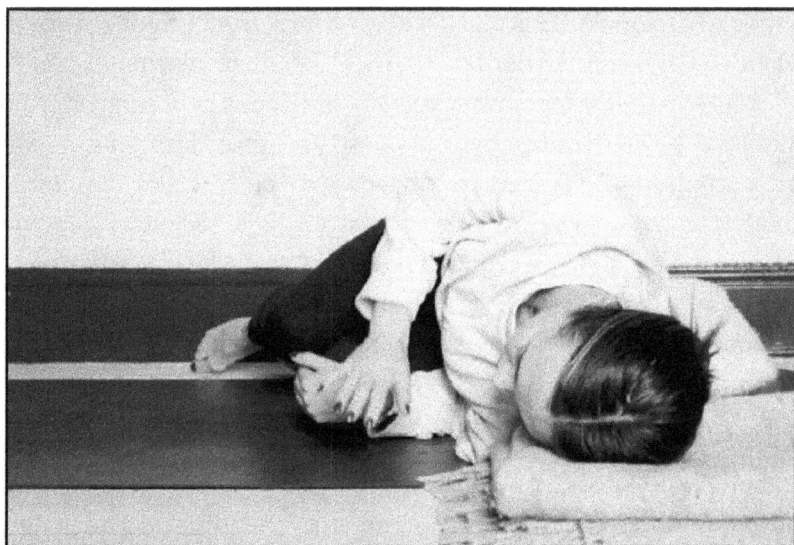

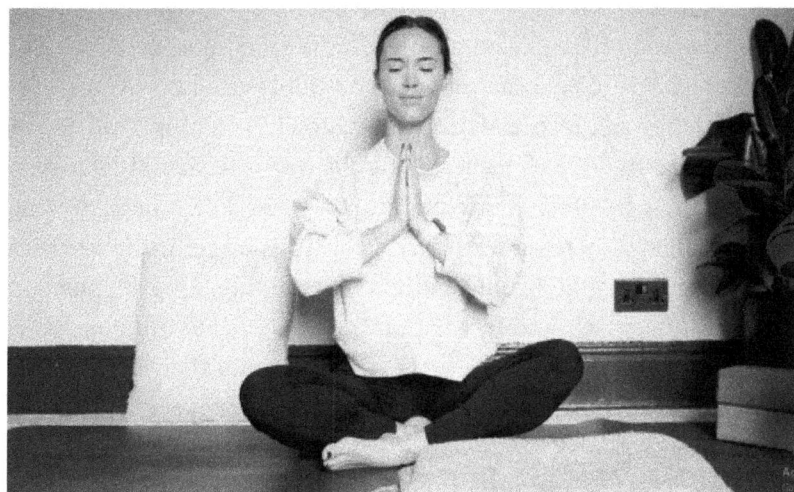

4.2 SOMATIC STRATEGIES FOR ALLEVIATING CHRONIC TENSION

Chronic tension can feel like a constant weight that never lifts. That persistent tightness in your muscles doesn't seem to go away, no matter what you do. This tension often comes from prolonged stress. When you're stressed, your body stays in a state of alertness, ready to react. Over time, this constant state of readiness wears on your muscles, causing them to become tense and sore. This tension isn't just uncomfortable; it can also impact your posture and movement. Another common cause of chronic stress is a sedentary lifestyle. Sitting for long hours, whether at work or home, can lead to stiffness, particularly in areas such as the shoulders, neck, and lower back. Without movement, your muscles don't get the chance to stretch and relax.

Somatic exercises provide a means to release the built-up tension. These exercises focus on gentle movements that help your muscles release tightness. Shoulder-release exercises are a great starting point. Sit or stand comfortably and roll your shoulders forward and backward. As you do this, pay attention to how your shoulders feel. This movement helps loosen the muscles and improve blood flow. Gentle neck stretches can also provide relief. Slowly tilt your head to one side, allowing the stretch to feel along the opposite side of your neck. Hold for a few breaths, then switch to the other side. These stretches ease tension and increase flexibility. Pelvic tilts target the lower back, which often bears the brunt of stress from sitting. Lie on your back with your knees bent and feet flat on the floor. Gently tilt your pelvis upward, flattening your back against the ground, then release. This movement can reduce lower back tension and improve mobility.

Practicing tension release exercises regularly offers long-term benefits. You'll notice increased flexibility and mobility as you incorporate these movements into your routine. Your muscles become more adaptable, making everyday activities more manageable and comfortable. These exercises also reduce pain and discomfort. By releasing tension, you allow your muscles to relax and heal. This, in turn, improves your overall sense of well-being. You may move more effi-ciently, and tasks that once seemed daunting become manageable. Regular practice creates a positive cycle where less tension leads to more movement, and more movement leads to less stress.

Creating a personalized tension-relief routine can help you address your specific needs. Start by identifying your personal tension hotspots. These are areas where you most often feel tightness or discomfort. It could be your neck, shoulders, or lower back. Once you've identified these areas, set daily goals for your tension-releasing exercises. This doesn't need to take hours. Even a few minutes each day can make a big difference. Consistency is key. Making these exer-cises a routine helps your body build resilience against tension. You can practice in the morning to start your day quickly or in the evening to unwind before bed. Find what works best for you and stick with it.

To make your routine effective, pay attention to how your body responds to each exercise—notice which movements feel good and which areas need more focus. Adjust your routine as necessary to meet your changing needs. Your body is unique, and your routine should reflect that. Over time, you may need to modify your exercises to keep them challenging and beneficial. This adaptability ensures that your practice continues to support your well-being.

4.3 EVENING ROUTINES TO UNWIND AND RELAX

As the day draws closer, the body craves a moment to unwind. Estab-lishing an evening routine can signal to the body that it's time to relax and prepare for sleep. The mind often races with thoughts from the day, making it hard to transition to rest. A calming routine acts like a gentle reminder to slow down. It tells your body to release the day's stresses. This transition from activity to rest is essential for the body and mind. It helps improve sleep quality, waking you up refreshed and ready for the day.

Evening routines can vary, but they often include soothing exercises that promote relaxation. Gentle yoga poses are a great way to unwind. These poses stretch the body, release tension, and ease the mind. Consider poses like the child's pose or legs-up-the-wall pose. They are simple yet effective in calming the body. Another way to transition into rest is through breathing exercises. These help clear the mind and reduce stress. Consider sitting quietly and taking slow, deep breaths. Please focus on the air filling your lungs and then releasing it. This simple practice can create a sense of peace and readiness for sleep.

The psychological benefits of evening routines extend beyond just helping you sleep. They can help reduce stress and anxiety levels. When you engage in calming activities, you let your mind detach from the day's worries. This detachment helps create a mental boundary between the stress of the day and the restful night ahead. It's like drawing a line in the sand, separating what was from what will be. This separation can lead to a more peaceful night's sleep and a more positive outlook on the new day.

Creating a personalized evening routine can make this time even more special. Think about what activities help you relax. It could be reading a favorite book, listening to soothing music, or meditating. These activities can become a cherished part of your evening. Tailor your routine to fit your needs and preferences. If you enjoy a hot bath, make it a ritual. Light some candles, add a few drops of essential oil, and unwind with a soothing soak. Or, if you prefer quiet moments, find a cozy spot to meditate or practice gratitude. Reflect on the day's positives to set a peaceful tone before bed.

An evening routine isn't about doing everything perfectly; it's about doing the right things at the right time. It's about creating a space that feels right for relaxation. Experiment with various activities until you find what works best for you. Be flexible and allow your routine to adapt to your changing needs. Some nights, you might spend more time in meditation. On other evenings, you might read or write in a journal. The key is consistency. When your body knows what to expect, it responds more readily. Over time, you'll notice the benefits. Your sleep will improve, stress will decrease, and you'll feel more balanced.

Alternate Nostril Breathing (Nadi Shodhana)

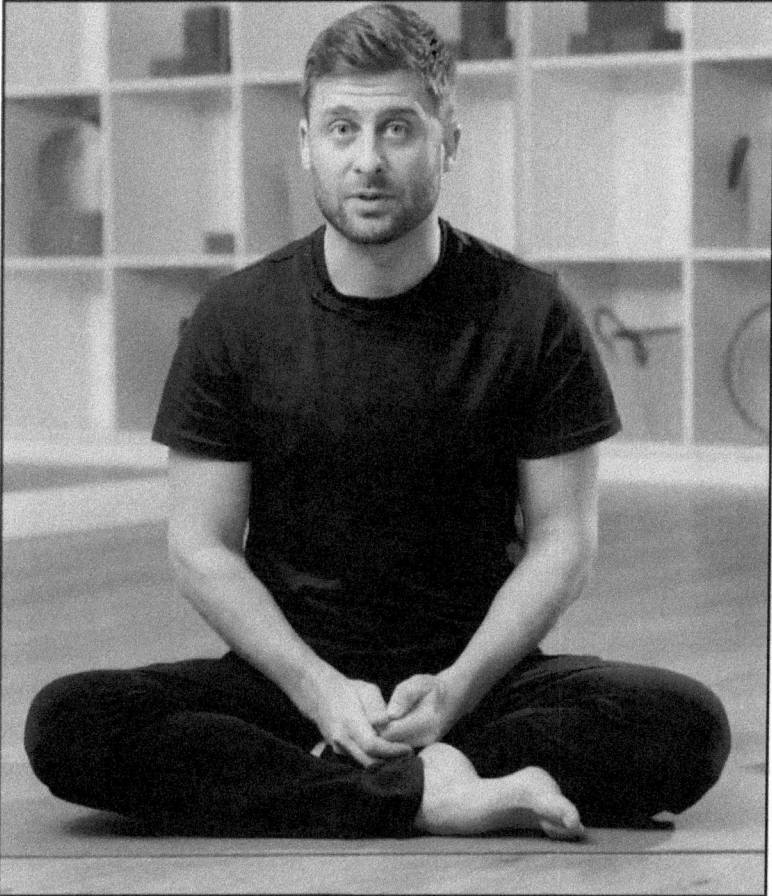

Sit comfortably and relax your shoulders.

Close your right nostril with your thumb, inhale through the left.

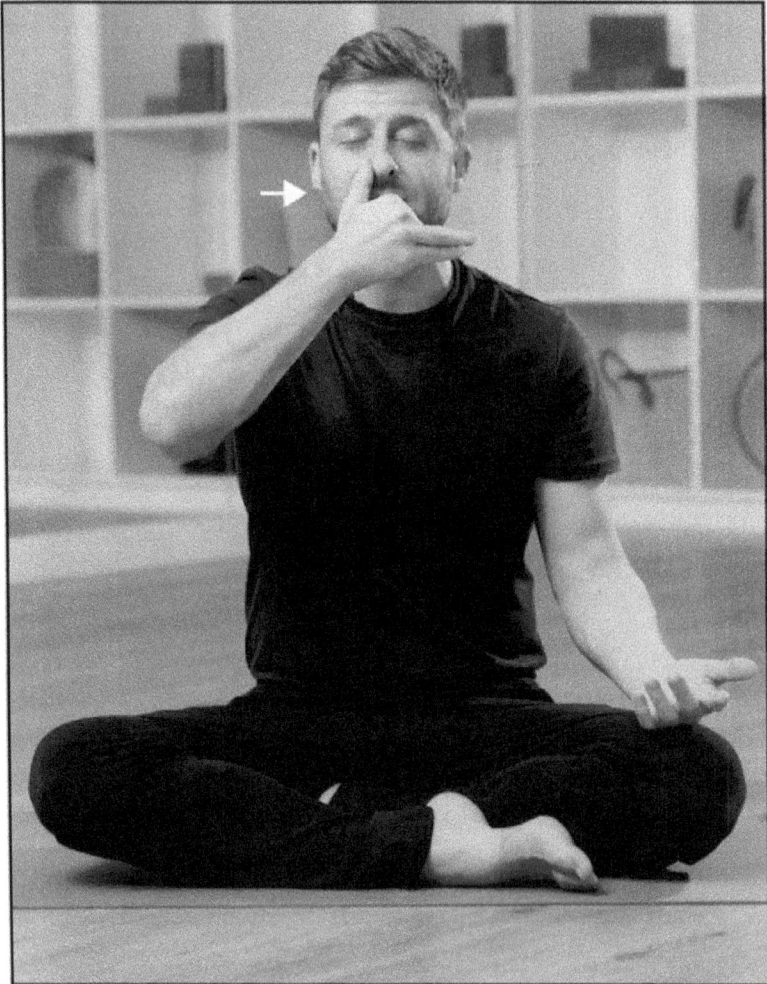

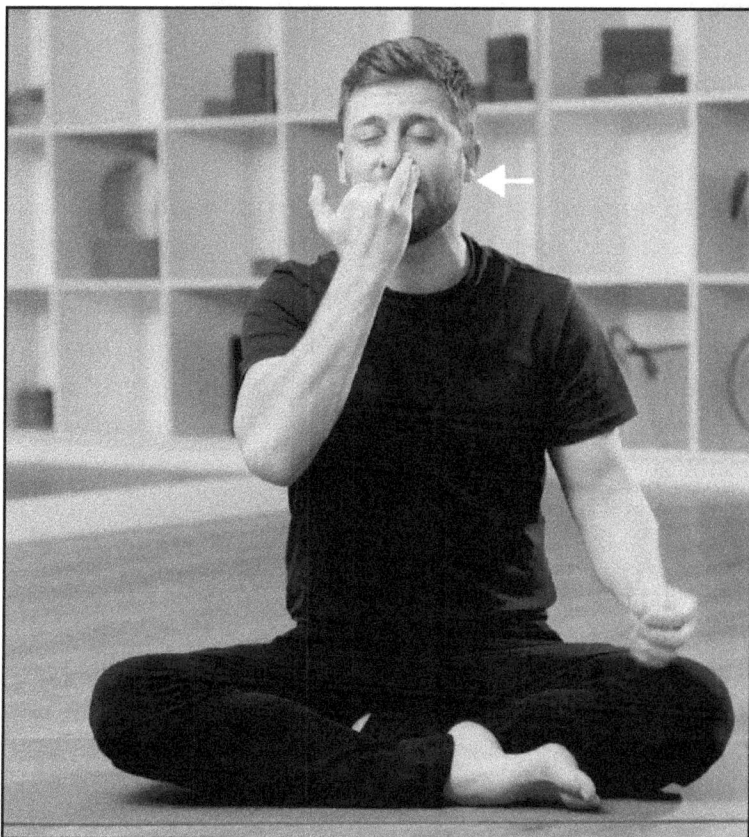

Close the left nostril with a finger, exhale through the right.

Inhale through the right, switch, and exhale through the left — repeat slowly for 4-6 rounds.

Sleep is crucial for our health and well-being, yet many of us struggle to get the rest we need. Insomnia and restless nights can leave you feeling drained and irritable. Somatic exercises provide a gentle approach to enhancing sleep quality by stimulating the body's relaxation response. When you practice these exercises, your body learns to release tension and stress, creating an ideal environment for sleep. This relaxation response calms your nervous system, making it easier to fall asleep and stay asleep through the night. By reducing physical tension, somatic exercises help to relax both the body and mind, paving the way for restful sleep.

One effective technique for better sleep is the body scan. This exercise guides your attention through each body part, helping you notice and release tension. Lie comfortably on your back, close your eyes, and take a few deep breaths. Begin by focusing on your toes, then gradually shift your attention upward through your legs, torso, arms, and head. As you focus on each area, imagine it becoming soft and relaxed. This practice calms your mind and prepares your body for sleep by easing muscle tension. Another helpful method is visualization. Picture a serene scene, such as a quiet beach or a tranquil forest. Imagine yourself there, feeling the warmth of the sun or the cool breeze. Visualization creates a sense of calm, helping you drift into a restful sleep.

The benefits of improved sleep extend beyond just feeling rested. When you sleep well, your mood improves, and you handle stress more effectively. A good night's sleep enhances cognitive function, making it easier to focus and solve problems more effectively. It boosts your immune system, helping your body fight off illness. With regular, quality sleep, you can experience increased energy and a positive outlook on life. These benefits underscore the importance of addressing sleep issues, and somatic exercises offer a straightforward and effective solution. Integrating these practices into your daily routine sets the stage for improved sleep and overall well-being.

Consider the story of Anna, who struggled with insomnia for years. She often lay awake for hours, her mind racing with worries and to-do lists. After learning about somatic exercises, Anna began practicing a nightly body scan. This simple exercise helped her mind settle and her body relax. Over time, her sleep improved, and she woke up feeling refreshed. Another person, John, used visualization to combat his restless nights. He envisioned a serene mountain scene, which calmed his thoughts and helped him drift off to sleep. These testimonials illustrate how somatic exercises transform sleep quality and improve daily life.

Incorporating somatic exercises into your bedtime routine can be a game-changer. Dedicating just a few minutes each night to these practices can create a robust foundation for restful sleep. This approach addresses sleep issues and promotes a deeper connection between your body and mind. As you continue to explore somatic exercises, you'll find that they offer more than just improved sleep. They enhance your well-being, helping you feel more balanced and at peace.

This chapter explores tools such as breathwork, grounding techniques, and somatic exercises to enhance relaxation and promote better sleep. Each practice offers a unique way to calm the mind and ease the body, setting the stage for restful nights and energized days. As we progress, we'll continue to build on these foundations, exploring ways to integrate these exercises into your life for better health and harmony.

CHAPTER 5

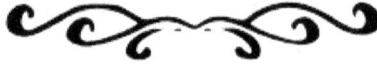

ENHANCING FLEXIBILITY
AND STRENGTH SAFELY

Picture yourself moving through the day with a grace that feels effortless. Your body flows from one task to the next without the familiar pull of tight muscles. This isn't a fantasy but an outcome you can achieve with gentle flow routines. These routines use smooth, continuous movements to enhance flexibility. Unlike static stretching, which involves holding a pose, gentle flow routines focus on dynamic movement. This approach enhances blood flow and increases muscle temperature, thereby preparing your body for increased activity.

Flow-based movement sequences are at the heart of these routines. Imagine a gentle wave rolling onto the shore, then retreating into the sea. This fluid motion is what you aim for in your exercises. You move with intention, flowing from one pose to another without pause. This kind of movement helps maintain your body's natural rhythm. It encourages your muscles to lengthen and contract smoothly, which improves flexibility and reduces the risk of injury. Dynamic stretching, which involves moving muscles and joints with sports-specific motions, is especially beneficial for warming up. It engages your body in a way that static stretching may not, according to the Cleveland Clinic (SOURCE 1).

Gentle flow routines enhance flexibility and improve overall well-being. When you practice these exercises regularly, you help your muscles stay supple and your joints mobile. This translates into better movement in daily life. Tasks like reaching for a high shelf or bending to tie your shoes become easier. This increase in joint mobility also results in reduced stiffness and discomfort. Over time, you'll notice reduced muscle tightness, often leading to greater comfort and ease in your movements.

One example of a gentle flow exercise is a sun salutation-inspired sequence. This series of movements mimics the rising and setting of the sun. You begin standing, reach the sky, and then fold forward. You transition into a plank, followed by a gentle backbend. Each movement flows into the next, creating a continuous cycle. This sequence stretches many body parts, including your arms, legs, and back. It helps improve flexibility and can be done at your own pace, adjusting to your body's needs.

Another effective exercise is the flowing spinal twist. This movement involves gently twisting your torso from side to side. You start by sitting or standing tall, then slowly rotate your upper body in one direction. Hold the twist for a moment, then return to the center. Repeat on the other side. This exercise helps release tension in your spine and improves flexibility. It also encourages fluidity in your movements, preventing injuries and enhancing your range of motion.

The importance of fluid movement cannot be overstated. When your movements are smooth, you reduce the strain on your muscles and joints. This fluidity helps prevent injury and allows you to move more freely. To achieve seamless transitions between poses, focus on your breath. As you inhale, prepare for the next movement. As you exhale, flow into the new pose. This synchronization between breath and movement encourages balance and harmony in your practice.

Regular practice of gentle flow routines has a lasting impact on your body. You build flexibility that supports your daily activities and overall health. This practice isn't just about stretching your body and creating a more flexible life; it's also about cultivating a more resilient mindset. By dedicating time to these exercises, you invest in yourself, setting the foundation for a life of ease and mobility.

Interactive Element: Try a Gentle Flow Routine

- **Sun Salutation Sequence**: Begin standing, reach up, fold forward, step back to plank, lower to a gentle backbend, and return to standing. Repeat slowly, focusing on the breath and smooth transitions.
- **Flowing Spinal Twist**: Sit or stand tall. Gently twist your torso to one side, hold, and then return to the center. Repeat on the other side. Aim for fluid, relaxed movements.

These gentle exercises offer a simple yet effective way to enhance flexibility. They invite you to explore your body's capabilities, encouraging a more fluid and graceful way of life.

5.1 SOMATIC TECHNIQUES FOR STRENGTH RECOVERY POST-INJURY

Imagine recovering from an injury and feeling uncertain about regaining your strength. It's a tough place to be, but somatic exercises can offer a gentle path to recovery. These exercises focus on low-impact movements, which are kind to the body as you heal. Instead of pushing your limits, you engage in movements that help rebuild muscle memory. This approach allows your body to remember how to move efficiently and safely. It supports your muscles as they relearn tasks that once seemed daunting. You gradually restore your strength through somatic exercises without adding stress to your healing body.

Rebuilding strength after an injury requires patience and the right exercises. Isometric exercises are a great starting point. These involve holding a position without moving, which helps build joint stability and strength. For example, try pressing your hands against a wall and holding the position. This activates muscles without straining them. Another effective method is using resistance bands. These bands provide controlled tension that helps strengthen muscles. You can perform simple exercises, such as bicep curls or leg presses. They allow you to adjust the resistance to match your current ability, making them ideal for recovery and improvement.

Gentle leg lifts are another valuable exercise for those recovering from lower-body injuries. Lie on your back with one leg bent and the other straight. Slowly lift the straight leg, hold for a moment, and lower it. This exercise strengthens your legs without stressing your joints. It also improves balance and coordination, aiding your recovery process. As you practice these exercises, you'll notice gradual improvements in strength and mobility. Each session builds upon the last, creating a foundation for a more substantial and resilient body.

Personalized recovery plans play a crucial role in effective healing. Every injury is unique, and so is your body. Tailoring your exercises based on your specific needs and limitations is essential. Consulting with healthcare professionals can help guide you in creating a personalized plan that aligns with your recovery goals. They can offer insights into which exercises are safe and beneficial for your condition. Their expertise ensures you avoid movements that might cause harm. By working with professionals, you gain confidence in your recovery path, knowing that you're supported by expert guidance.

The psychological benefits of recovery through somatic practices are significant. As you engage in these exercises, you boost your confidence and mental resilience. Overcoming physical limitations empowers you, showing you that progress is possible. Many individuals have shared their stories of successful recovery, highlighting the impact of somatic exercises on their well-being. One person, for instance, spoke about regaining strength after a knee injury. Through consistent practice, they were able to return to activities they loved. Another shared how somatic exercises helped them feel more in tune with their body, reducing anxiety about re-injury.

These testimonials demonstrate the transformative power of somatic exercises. They indicate that recovery is not just about physical healing, but also about emotional resilience. As you rebuild your body, you also rebuild your confidence. This newfound resilience extends beyond your recovery, influencing other areas of your life. You become more aware of your body's signals, learning to trust its abilities. This awareness fosters a deeper connection with yourself, promoting long-term well-being and overall happiness.

5.2 BUILDING CORE STRENGTH WITH MINDFUL MOVEMENTS

Think of your core as the sturdy trunk of a tree, supporting the limbs and branches that reach out in all directions. A strong core is vital for maintaining overall physical health and stability. It plays a crucial role in posture, helping you stand tall and move with confidence. Your core muscles, which include the abdominals, obliques, and lower back, work together to stabilize your body. This stability is crucial for balance. It helps prevent falls and keeps your movements precise and controlled. A strong core also acts as a natural brace, protecting your spine and reducing the risk of injury during everyday activities. When your core is strong, your body can handle more physical stress, whether you're lifting a heavy bag or twisting to reach something on a high shelf.

Mindful exercises can effectively build core strength while engaging both body and mind. One such exercise is the plank, known for its simplicity and effectiveness. You engage multiple core muscles by holding your body in a straight line from head to heels. Plank variations, such as side or forearm planks, add variety and challenge. Focus on your breath as you hold each position. Inhale deeply and exhale slowly, using your breath to maintain stability. This awareness helps you stay present and enhances the effectiveness of the exercise. Another mindful exercise is the seated Russian twist. Sit with your knees bent and lean back slightly. Hold your hands together and twist your torso from side to side, engaging your core. Breathe in as you return to the center and out as you twist. This movement strengthens your obliques and improves rotational stability.

Pelvic tilts are another simple yet powerful exercise. Lie on your back with your knees bent and feet flat. Gently tilt your pelvis upward, flattening your lower back against the floor. Hold for a few seconds, then release. Focus on the movement and your breathing. This exercise targets the lower abdominals and supports the spine. It promotes awareness of how your core contributes to overall posture and balance. Regular mindful movements can lead to a stronger, more resilient core.

Gradual progression is key when building core strength. It's essential to increase exercise intensity slowly to prevent strain. Begin with comfortable exercises and gradually increase the repetitions or hold positions for more extended periods. Pay attention to how your body responds. If an exercise causes discomfort, adjust it to suit your current level of ability. Avoid pushing yourself too hard, too soon. This approach helps prevent injuries and ensures that your progress is sustainable and long-lasting. Over time, you'll notice improvements in your core strength and overall stability.

Breathing plays a crucial role in core exercises. It acts as a bridge between mind and body, enhancing the impact of each movement. By controlling your breath, you can increase the effectiveness of your exercises. Focus on synchronizing your breath with your movements. For instance, inhale during the preparation phase of an exercise and exhale during the exertion phase. This rhythm supports core engagement and helps stabilize your body. Controlled breathing also promotes relaxation, reducing tension in other parts of the body. Incorporating breath awareness into your practice creates a more mindful and holistic approach to strengthening your core.

Incorporating mindful core exercises into your routine can transform how you move and feel. They enhance your posture, improve your balance, and reduce the risk of injury. These exercises invite you to explore your body's potential, encouraging a deeper connection between mind and body. With time and consistency, you'll discover the benefits of a strong, stable core. It supports you in all aspects of life, from daily tasks to more demanding physical activities. As you progress, you'll find that this newfound strength enhances your overall sense of well-being, empowering you to move with greater confidence and ease.

Gentle Flow Sun Salutation

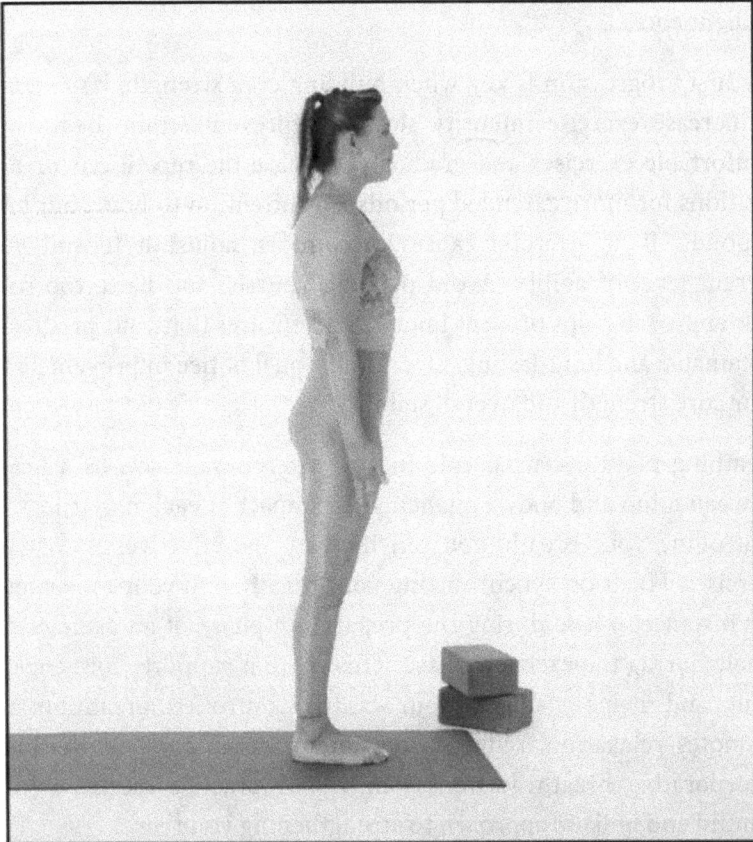

- Stand tall with feet together or hip-width apart.

- Let your hands rest freely by your side.

- Take a grounding breath to begin.

- Reach through the fingertips and gently arch back, lifting your heart.

- Inhale and raise your arms overhead.

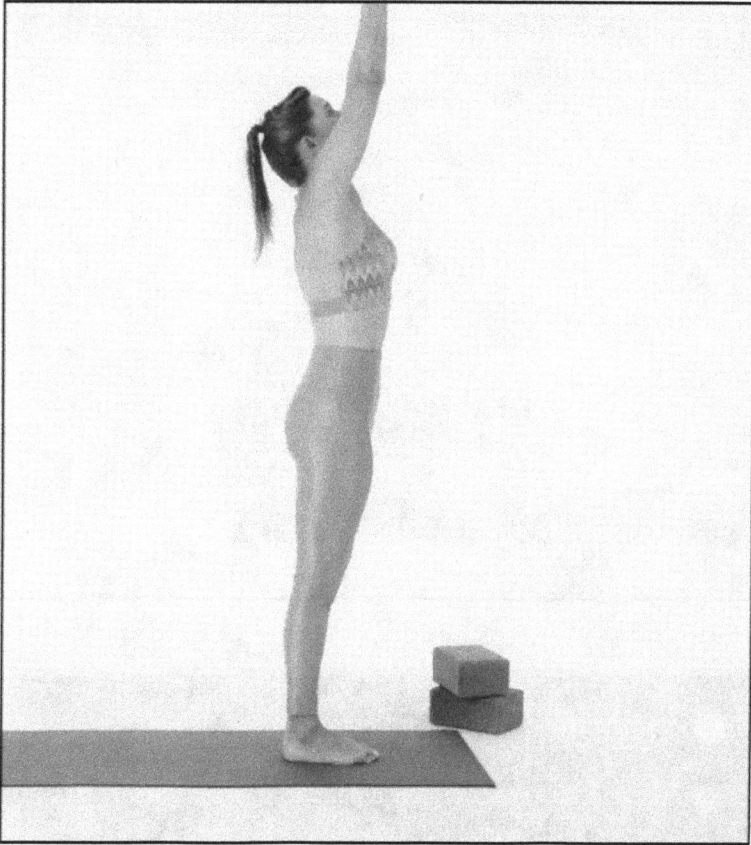

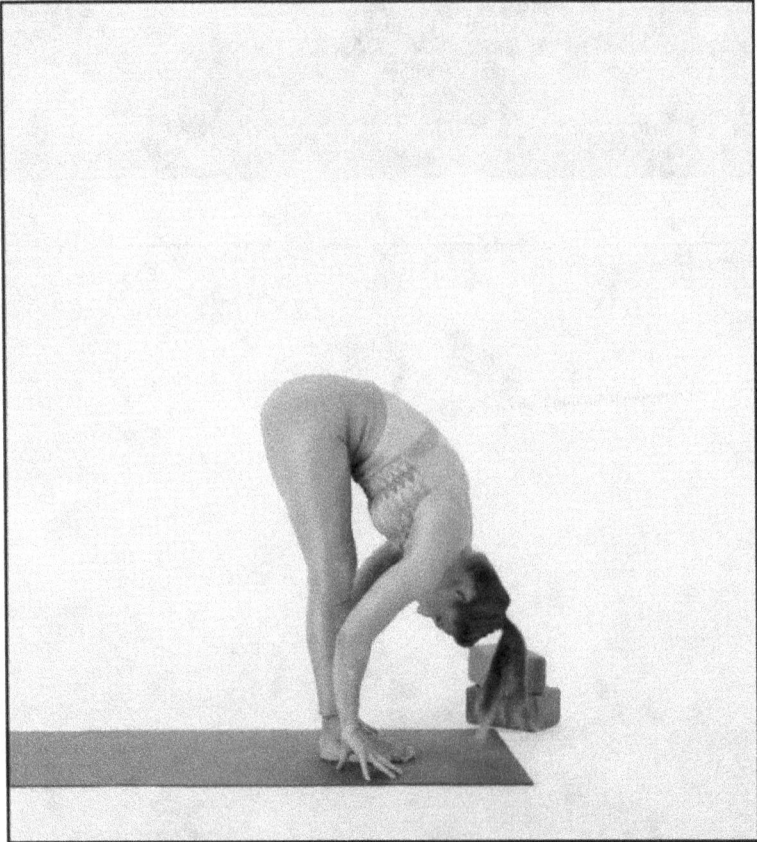

- Exhale and fold forward from your hips.

- Bend your knees slightly if needed to avoid strain.

- Let your head and neck relax.

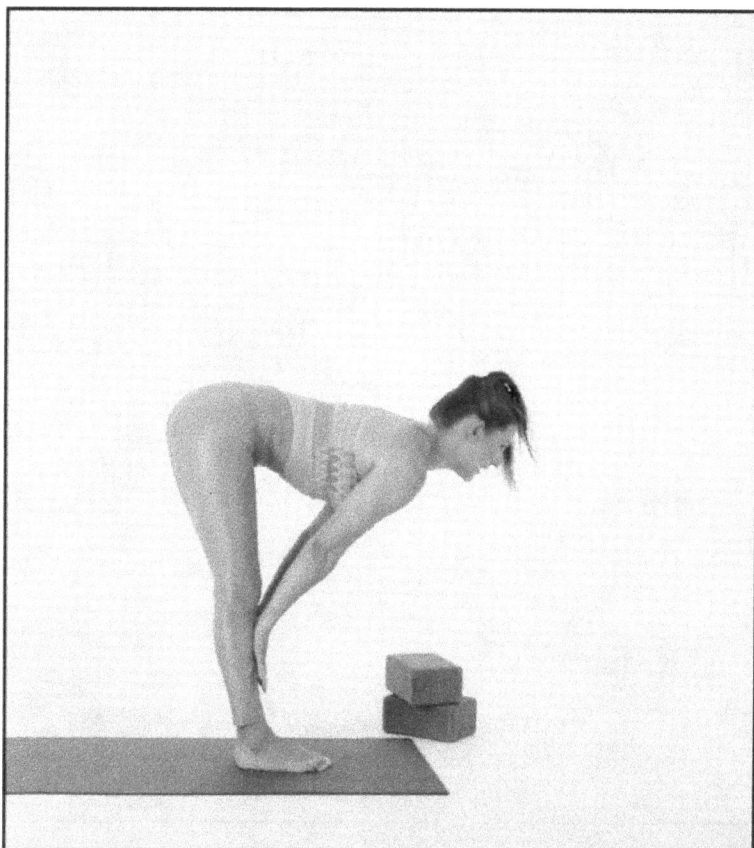

- Inhale and lift your chest halfway up.
- Place your hands on your shins or fingertips on the mat.
- Lengthen your spine forward.

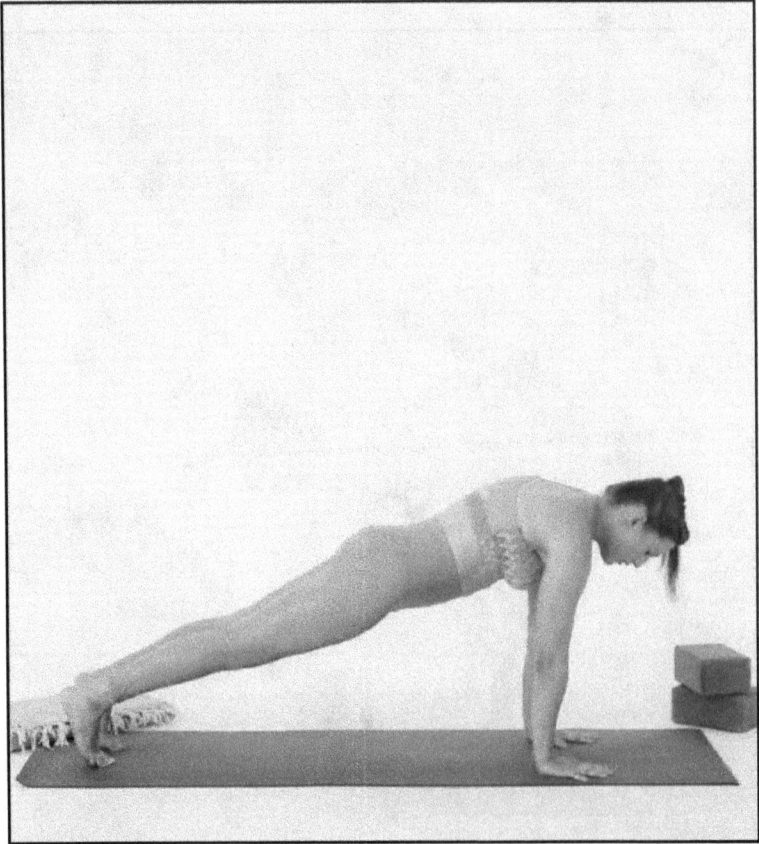

- Exhale and place your hands firmly on the mat.

- Step both feet back into a high plank position.

- Engage your core and keep your body in one straight line.

- Lower down on an exhale — either knees-chest-chin (gentle) or through full chaturanga.

- Elbows stay close to your sides.

- Hover above the mat or come all the way to the floor.

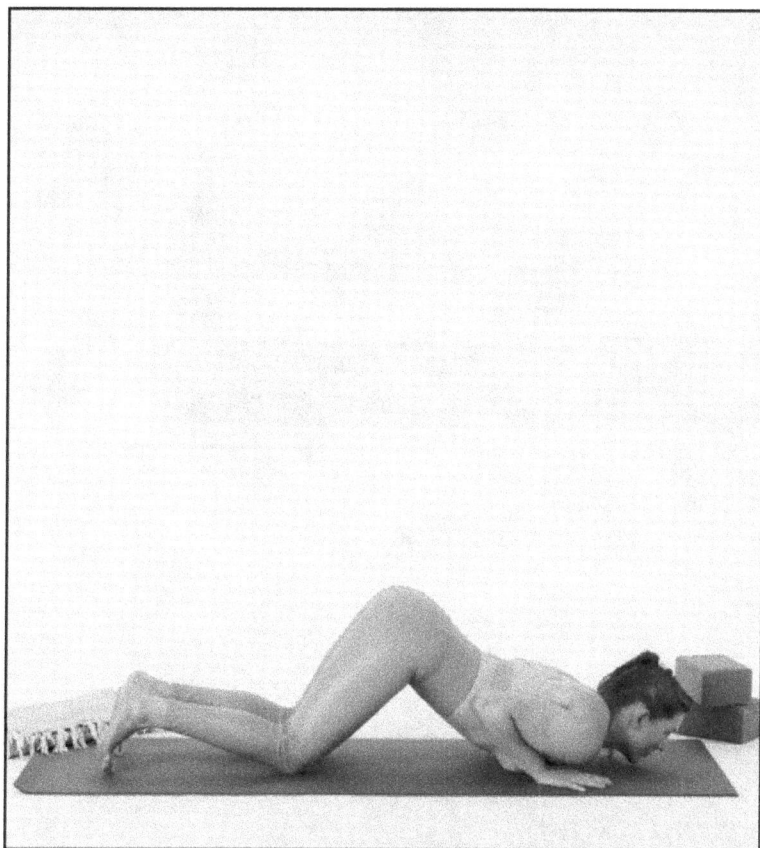

- Inhale and slide forward, lifting your chest.

- Press into your hands, straighten your arms, and open your heart.

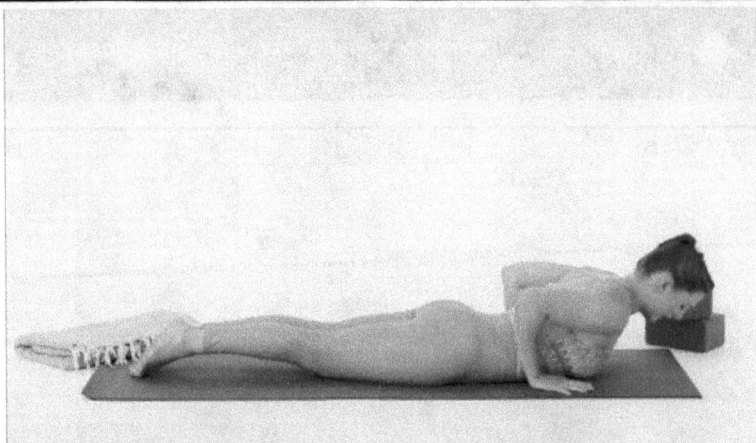

- Legs lift off the floor if you're in full Upward Dog.

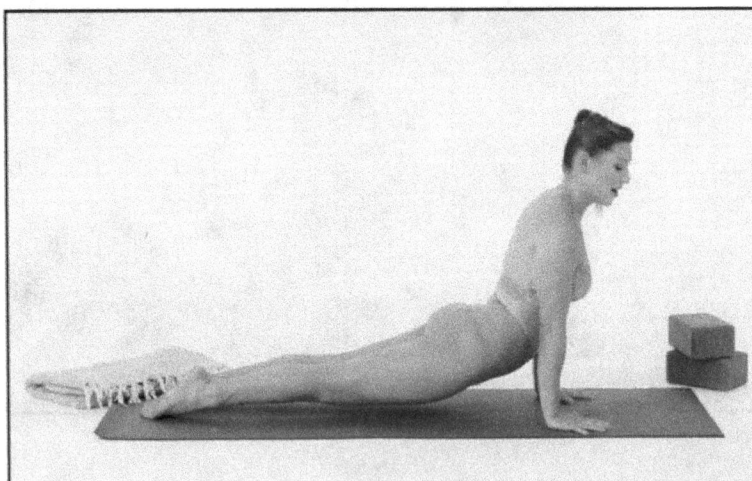

Exhale and lift your hips up and back.

Form an inverted V-shape with your body.

Feet are hip-width apart, hands shoulder-width.

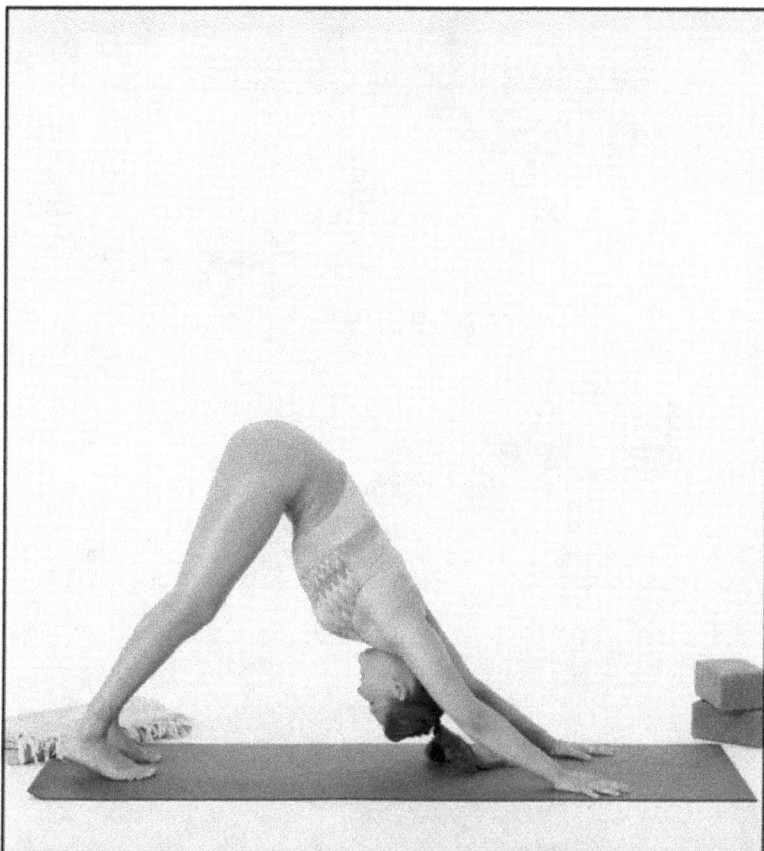

Hold for 3–5 breaths.

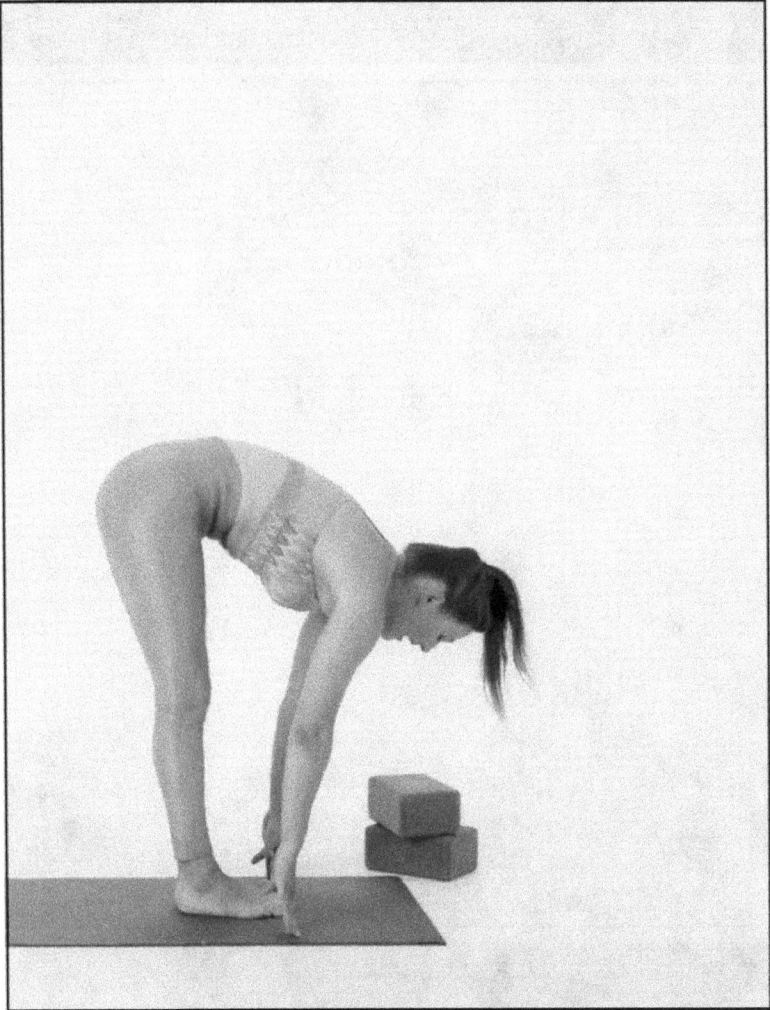

86

Inhale and lift your chest halfway, lengthening your spine.

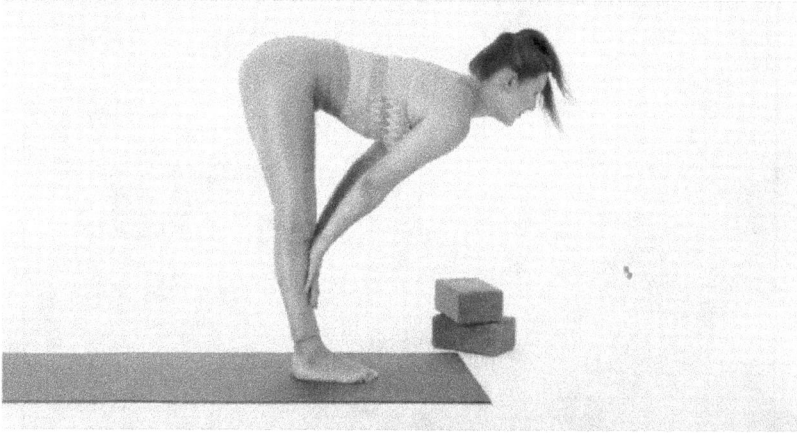

Exhale and release into the full forward fold.

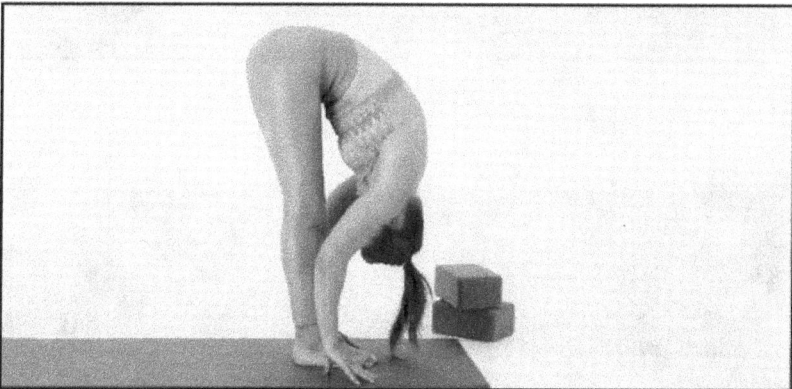

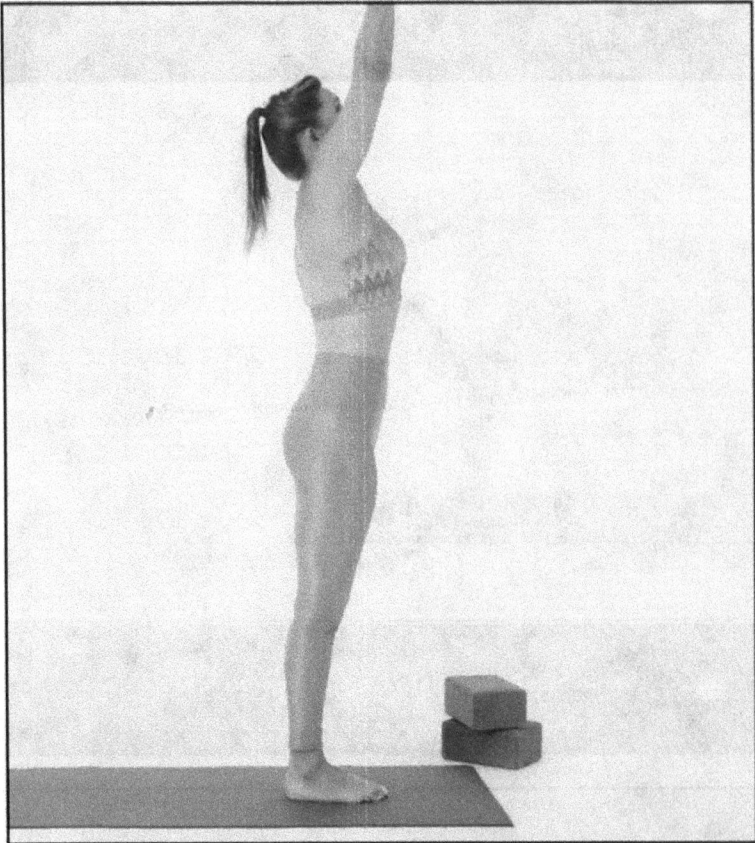

- Inhale, rise all the way up with arms overhead.
- Slight backbend if comfortable.

5.3 EXERCISES FOR BALANCE AND ALIGNMENT

Balance and alignment are two key elements that are vital to how efficiently you move throughout your day. They help you maintain stability, reduce the risk of falls, and support your body's structural integrity. When considering balance, think about how it impacts your daily activities. Whether standing in line, climbing stairs, or carrying groceries, balance keeps you upright and steady. Conversely, proper alignment ensures that your body is in the best position to function without strain. It helps prevent injuries, as misalignment can lead to unnecessary stress on your muscles and joints.

To improve these aspects, consider incorporating specific exercises into your routine. The tree pose is a classic exercise that enhances balance and stability. Stand on one leg and place the sole of your other foot against the inner thigh of your standing leg. Please keep your hands together at your chest or raise them overhead. Focus on a point in front of you to maintain your balance and stability. This pose strengthens your legs and core while improving your balance. Another effective exercise is the alignment-focused lunge. Step forward with one foot, bending both knees to lower your hips. Keep your back straight and your front knee aligned over your ankle. This movement promotes proper alignment and works your thighs and glutes. Balancing on one leg with mindful focus also helps. Stand tall and lift one foot off the ground. Hold this position while engaging your core and focusing on your balance. Switch legs after a few seconds. This exercise improves your balance and awareness of your body's posture.

Somatic focus adds an essential dimension to these exercises. You can enhance your balance and alignment by paying close attention to how your body feels. Notice where your weight is distributed and how your muscles engage. This awareness helps correct any misalignments and enhances your ability to hold each pose. Techniques for maintaining focus during balance exercises include keeping your gaze steady and using your breath to stay grounded. Inhale as you find your balance and exhale to deepen your focus. This connection between breath and movement enhances your stability and concentration.

Incorporating balance exercises into your daily routine requires little time or equipment. You can practice balance while brushing your teeth. Stand on one leg and focus on your posture as you brush your teeth. This simple practice turns a routine task into a moment for balance training. Another tip is to practice balancing while waiting for your coffee to brew or your toast to pop. These short exercises fit seamlessly into your day, making it easy to improve your balance without carving out extra time.

The benefits of regular balance and alignment training extend beyond physical health. As you become more balanced, you gain confidence in your movements. You feel more secure in your body, knowing that you can rely on it to support you. This confidence spills over into other areas of life, enhancing your overall well-being. When your body is aligned correctly, energy flows more freely, which reduces tension and fatigue. You move through your day efficiently, feeling connected and in tune with your body.

Balance and alignment exercises provide a pathway to enhanced movement and improved health. They encourage you to listen to your body and make minor, significant, impactful adjustments. As you practice, you'll notice changes in your movement and sensation. Your balance will improve, and your posture will become more refined. These simple yet powerful exercises provide a foundation for a more balanced and aligned life.

5.4 OVERCOMING LIMITED MOBILITY WITH SOMATIC PRACTICES

Life can take unexpected turns, and sometimes, mobility becomes an issue. Due to age or a sedentary lifestyle, limited mobility can impact your quality of life. It might be the stiffness in your knees when you get up or the struggle to reach for something on a high shelf. These challenges can make daily tasks frustrating and tiring. But there's hope. Somatic practices provide a gentle and effective way to improve your range of motion. They focus on movements that can be done even if you're sitting down. These exercises help you regain some of the freedom that mobility issues have taken away.

Chair yoga is one such practice that can make a huge difference. You don't need to stand or move much to benefit from it. Sitting comfortably in a chair, you can do various poses that stretch your arms, legs, and back. It helps improve circulation and flexibility, making your body feel more open and relaxed. These movements are gentle, yet they provide enough engagement to boost your mobility. They allow you to explore your body's capabilities without overexerting yourself.

Gentle upper-body stretches are another option. If you've spent hours at a desk or in front of the TV, your shoulders and neck might feel tight. Simple stretches can ease this tension. While sitting, you can raise your arms overhead, then bring them down, feeling the stretch flow through your shoulders. You can also tilt your head to each side, stretching the muscles in your neck. These small actions may seem minor, but they can have a significant impact on how you feel.

Modified Tai Chi offers a solution for those who prefer a more flowing movement. This ancient practice involves slow, deliberate motions that promote balance and coordination. Modified versions of Tai Chi are suitable for seniors or anyone with limited mobility. The gentle movements focus on shifting weight from one foot to the other. This practice promotes body awareness and helps improve mobility in a safe and controlled manner.

Adaptability is key when it comes to somatic practices. Everyone's body is different, and what works for one person might not work for another. Listening to your body and adjusting exercises to fit your needs is essential. Modify the movement or try a different exercise if something doesn't feel right. Your body will signal what it needs, and paying attention to these signals is crucial. This approach ensures that your practice remains supportive and beneficial.

Many people have found success in enhancing their mobility through somatic exercises. Take Mary, for instance. She was a retiree who found it increasingly difficult to move freely. After incorporating chair yoga into her routine, she noticed a marked improvement. She could move more quickly and even regain some independence. Another person, John, used modified Tai Chi to manage his mobility issues. He discovered that the gentle movements helped him feel more stable and confident. These stories demonstrate that change is possible, even when it seems impossible.

As you explore these somatic practices, you'll find they offer more than just physical benefits. They provide a sense of empowerment and control over your body. This empowerment can boost your confidence and improve your overall outlook on life. You begin to realize that mobility limitations don't have to define you. With patience and consistency, you can improve your range of motion and enjoy a fuller, more active life.

Resistance Band Seated Row

- Sit on the floor with your legs extended straight out in front of you.

- Loop a resistance band around your feet and hold the ends in both hands.

- Keep your spine upright and core engaged.

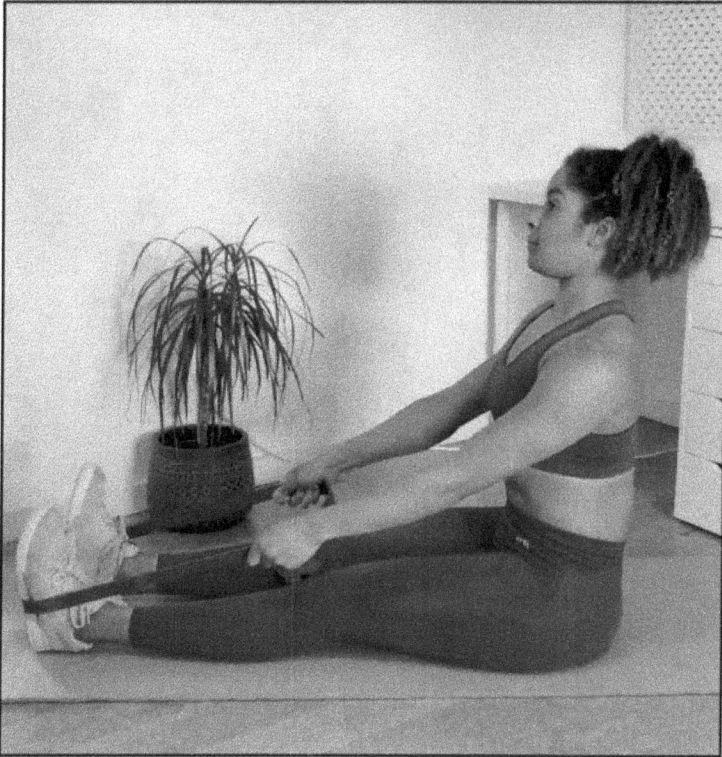

- Exhale as you pull the band toward your torso, bending your elbows back.

- Squeeze your shoulder blades together gently.

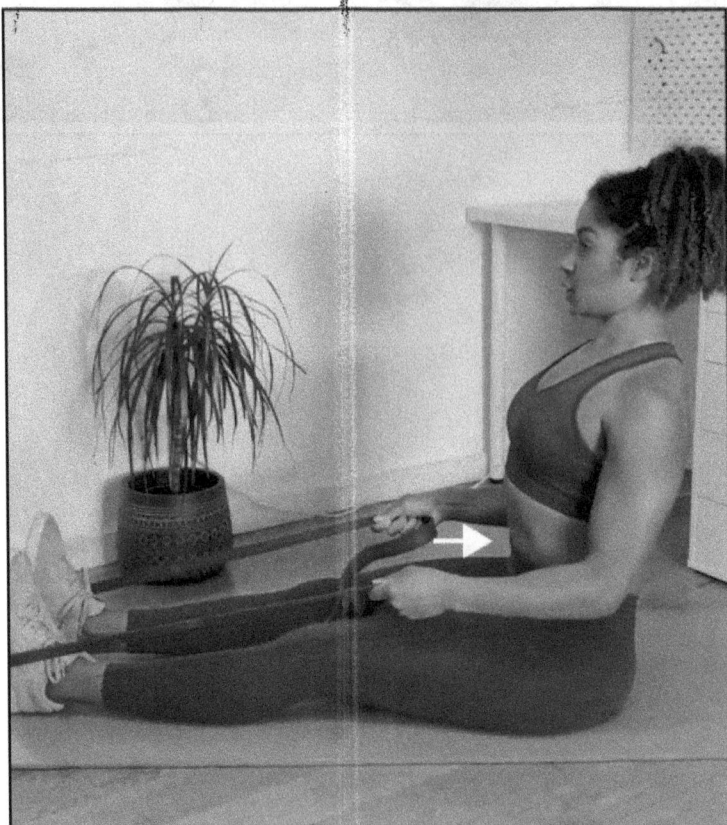

Inhale as you return your arms to the starting position with control.

Keep your posture steady.

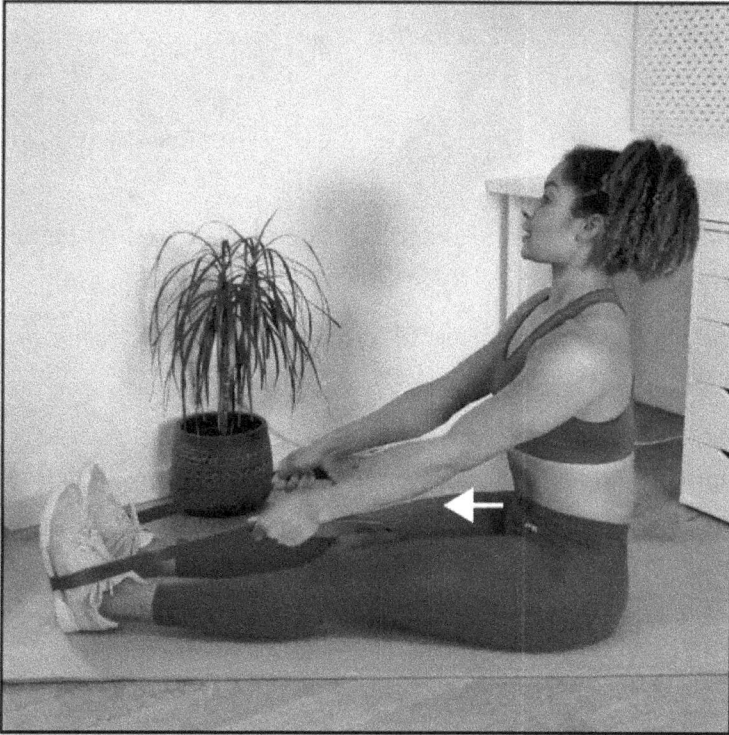

Repeat 8-12 times.

Focus on smooth motion and steady breath.

MAKE A DIFFERENCE
WITH YOUR REVIEW

UNLOCK THE POWER OF GENEROSITY

"The best way to find yourself is to lose yourself in the service of others."

— MAHATMA GANDHI

People who give without expecting anything in return often live calmer, happier lives. So, let's make a difference together!

Would you help someone just like you—curious about *somatic therapy exercises* but unsure where to start?

My mission is to make **At Home Somatic Therapy Exercises for Beginners: Easy & Gentle Movements for Nervous System Regulation, Emotional Healing and Lasting Calm** simple, practical, and calming for everyone.

But to reach more people, I need your help.

Most people choose books based on reviews. So, I'm asking you to help a fellow beginner by leaving a review.

It costs nothing and takes less than a minute, but it could change someone's journey with somatic therapy. Your review could help...

- one more person ease stress at the end of a long day.
- one more beginner finally feel confident starting simple exercises.
- one more reader discover peace in their body and mind.
- one more person reduce tension and improve their sleep.
- one more step toward making somatic therapy accessible to everyone.

To make a difference, simply scan the QR code below or visit this link
to leave a review:

https://www.amazon.com/review/review-your-purchases/?asin=
B0G4JFRSC2

If you love helping others, you're my kind of person.

Thank you from the bottom of my heart!

S.C. Monroe

CHAPTER 6

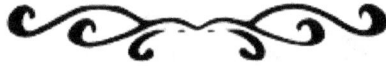

INCORPORATING MIND-BODY CONNECTION INTO DAILY LIFE

Picture this: you're in the middle of your daily routine, perhaps washing dishes or walking to your car, and instead of rushing through, you pause. You notice the feel of the water on your hands or the rhythm of your footsteps. This pause is more than just a moment of reflection; it is an entry point into mindful movement. The conscious movement combines the art of being present with the act of moving. It invites you to focus on your actions and the sensations in your body. Doing so transforms ordinary tasks into opportunities for awareness and relaxation. This practice can enhance body awareness and reduce stress, making it a simple yet powerful tool for everyday life.

Mindful movement is about being fully present and aware during routine activities. It involves paying attention to your body and surroundings without judgment or criticism. This awareness helps you connect with your body and can lead to a greater sense of peace. When you practice mindful movement, you engage with your body's sensations and the environment around you. This engagement fosters a deeper connection between mind and body, promoting mental and physical health. The benefits include improved focus, reduced stress, and increased relaxation. Being present allows you to turn mundane activities into moments of calm and clarity.

Incorporating mindfulness into daily tasks is easier than you think. Consider walking meditation during your daily commute. As you walk, focus on the sensations in your feet—a gentle heel-to-toe motion, the texture of the ground, or the rhythm of your steps. This focus can transform a routine walk into a moving meditation, fostering a sense of calm and presence. Another example is mindful dishwashing. Instead of rushing through the task, pay attention to the warmth of the water, the scent of the soap, and the texture of the dishes. Engage your senses fully, allowing the task to become a meditative experience. This practice will enable you to find peace every day and can turn ordinary chores into moments of mindfulness.

The impact of mindful movement on stress levels is significant. Grounding yourself in the present moment helps decrease stress and increase relaxation. Research suggests that mindfulness practices can help alleviate stress and improve emotional well-being. When you're mindful, you break the cycle of anxiety and worry, allowing yourself to relax and recharge. This break from stress can improve your mood and enhance your overall well-being. Incorporating mindful movement into your routine creates calm spaces that help balance the demands of daily life.

Finding creative opportunities for mindful movement can enrich your practice. Look for less apparent activities where you can incorporate mindfulness. For example, try mindful stretching while waiting in line. Instead of scrolling through your phone, take a moment to stretch your arms and shoulders. Focus on how your muscles feel and the sensation of the stretch. Another idea is engaging with nature through mindful gardening. As you tend to your plants, notice the texture of the soil, the sound of leaves rustling, and the colors around you. This practice deepens your connection to nature and enhances your sense of presence.

Interactive Element: Mindful Movement Challenge

- **Day 1**: Practice walking meditation during your commute. Focus on your breath and the sensations of walking.
- **Day 2**: Turn dishwashing into a mindful activity by engaging your senses.
- **Day 3**: Perform mindful stretching while waiting in line. Pay attention to the sensations in your body.
- **Day 4**: Spend time in the garden, focusing on the sensory experience.

Mindful movement doesn't require extra time or effort. It's about shifting your focus to the present, allowing each action to become a moment of awareness. This shift can bring about significant changes in your life. By embracing mindful movement, you enhance your body awareness, reduce stress, and find more joy in everyday tasks.

Walking Meditation

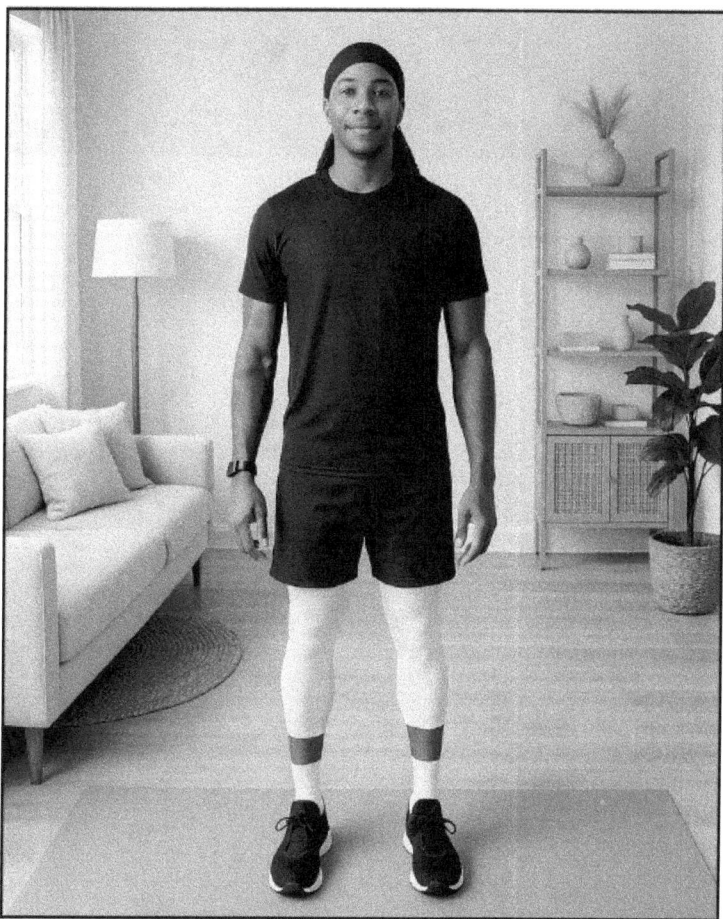

- Stand still for a moment before walking.

- Notice your breath and how your   feet feel on the ground.

Take slow, deliberate steps — lifting one foot, moving it forward, and placing it down with awareness.

Feel the heel-to-toe movement.

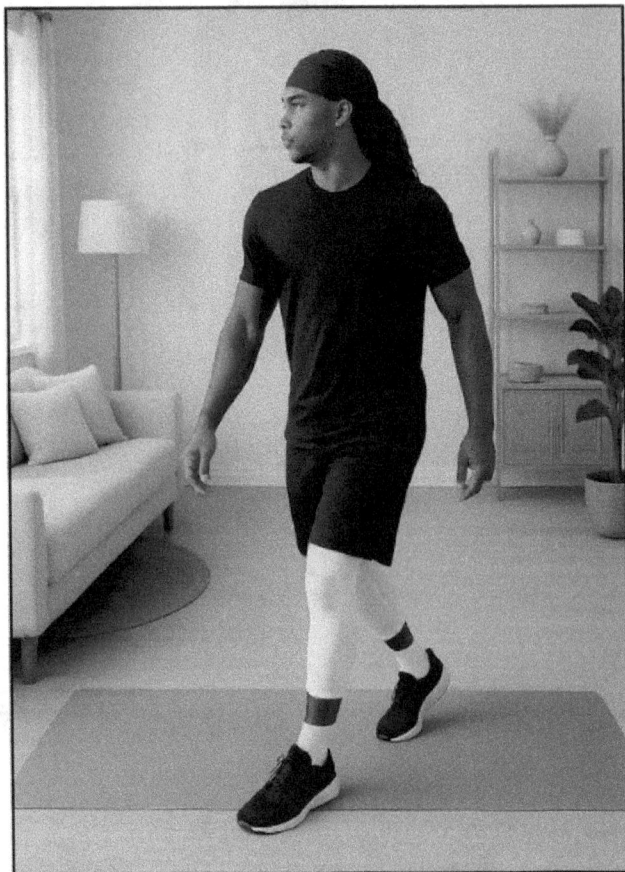

- With each step, mentally note: "lifting, moving, placing."
- Keep your breath soft and your awareness on your body and surroundings.

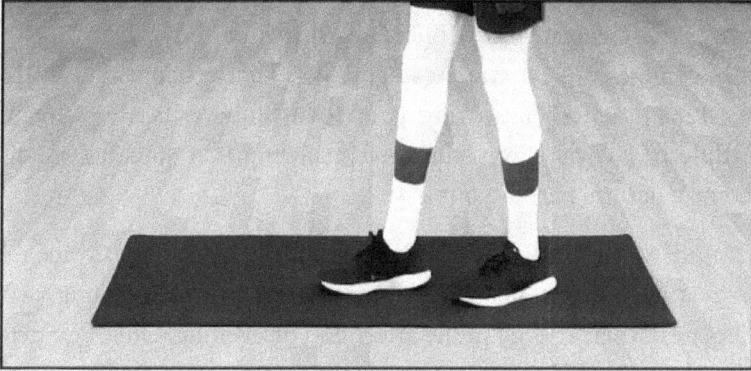

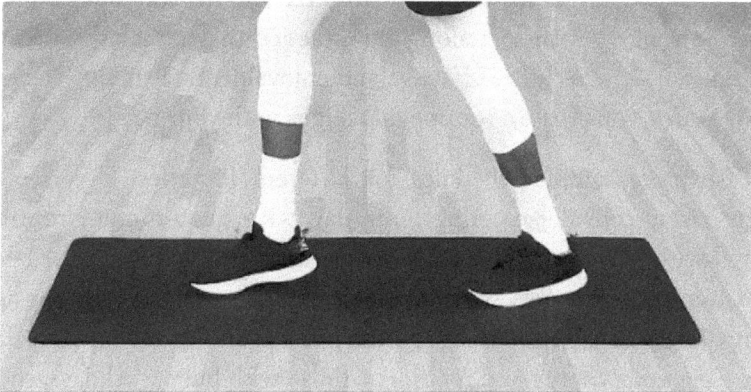

- When finished, pause briefly, take one slow breath, and acknowledge your body.

6.1 CREATING A DAILY SOMATIC PRACTICE SCHEDULE

Incorporating a structured routine can significantly enhance your experience with somatic exercises. Consistency is key. It enhances your commitment and maximizes the benefits of your practice. When you integrate these exercises into your daily life, they become as routine as brushing your teeth. This repetition helps build muscle memory and deepen your connection with your body. Over time, you notice changes in how you move and feel. These changes result from consistent practice, improving your focus and resilience. A regular schedule helps you stay committed, ensuring that somatic exercises become a natural part of your day.

To build a personalized schedule, start by identifying your peak energy times. Some people feel most alert in the morning, while others peak their energy in the afternoon or evening. Once you determine when you feel most energized, allocate time blocks for different types of exercises. For example, you might set aside mornings for gentle stretching and evenings for relaxation techniques. This approach allows you to tailor your practice to your body's natural rhythms, making it more effective and enjoyable. By listening to your body's cues, you create a routine that aligns with your needs.

Let's explore sample schedules for different lifestyles. If you're an early riser, consider starting your day with a 15-minute routine. Begin with a few minutes of focused breathing to wake up your body and mind. Follow this with gentle stretches to release any tension from the night. This morning routine sets a positive tone for your day, boosting your energy and focus. For those with busy workdays, short evening practices can help you unwind and relax. After dinner, spend 10 minutes on exercises that promote relaxation. Focus on slow, deep breathing and movements that soothe your muscles. This evening practice helps you release the day's stress, preparing you for restful sleep.

Spreading exercises throughout the day can help maintain your energy and focus. Consider incorporating a midday energy boost.

Find a quiet space where you can practice for five minutes. Engage in light stretching or deep breathing to recharge your mind and body. This brief break can enhance your concentration and productivity for the remainder of the day. Evening wind-down routines are also beneficial for better sleep. Before bed, spend a few minutes stretching your back and legs to help you relax. Pair these stretches with calming breathwork to signal your body that it's time to relax. This routine can help enhance sleep quality, leading to more restful nights and energized mornings.

Integrating these practices into your routine supports your physical and emotional health. A structured schedule helps you stay on track, making it easier to commit to regular practice. Over time, these exercises become a natural part of your life, enhancing your well-being. They offer a simple and effective way to connect with your body, reduce stress, and improve your overall quality of life.

6.2 ENHANCING ROUTINE ACTIVITIES WITH SOMATIC AWARENESS

Imagine feeling genuinely connected to your body in everything you do, from sitting at your desk to preparing a meal. This connection is the essence of somatic awareness. It involves tuning into your body's sensations and movements during everyday activities. You can enhance your overall well-being by paying attention to how your body feels. Body awareness helps you notice tension, fatigue, or other signals your body sends. This awareness is crucial in daily life because it guides you to make adjustments that promote comfort and health. When you're aware of your posture and movements, you can reduce strain and prevent discomfort. This practice fosters a more balanced and harmonious relationship with your body, thereby enhancing both your mental and physical health.

Think about how you sit at your desk. Often, we slouch or hunch over without realizing it. Conscious posture adjustments can make a big difference. Take a moment to notice how you're sitting. Are your shoulders tense? Is your back straight? You can ease tension and improve your posture by making minor adjustments, such as rolling your shoulders back or sitting up straighter. This simple practice can prevent long-term issues like back pain. Breathing exercises during meal preparation offer another opportunity for somatic awareness. As you cook, focus on taking slow, deep breaths. Feel your chest rise and fall. This calms your mind and helps you stay present, turning a routine task into a moment of relaxation and mindfulness.

The benefits of incorporating somatic awareness into daily tasks are significant. Paying attention to your body can enhance your focus and reduce stress. This increased awareness allows you to respond to your body's needs more quickly. For example, if you feel tension building, you can take a moment to stretch or adjust your posture. This practice leads to increased productivity and concentration. When your body is comfortable and relaxed, your mind can focus better on the task. You become more efficient in your work and daily activities, experiencing less mental fatigue. This heightened focus can improve your performance and overall satisfaction with your accomplishments.

To maintain somatic awareness throughout the day, consider setting reminders to help you stay focused and mindful. These can be simple prompts to check in with your body, like an alarm on your phone or a sticky note on your computer. When the reminder goes off, pause and take a moment to notice how you feel. Are you holding tension anywhere? Is your breathing shallow? Use this time to make any necessary adjustments. Journaling your experiences of heightened awareness can also be helpful. Please take a few minutes each day to write down what you notice about your body and how you respond to it. This practice encourages reflection and growth. It helps you track your progress and identify patterns in your body's feelings. Over time, you'll become more attuned to your body's signals, leading to improved well-being and a deeper connection with yourself.

Desk or Chair Somatic Check-In

- Sit upright in your chair with both feet flat on the floor.

- Rest your hands on your lap or desk.

- Take one slow, steady breath.

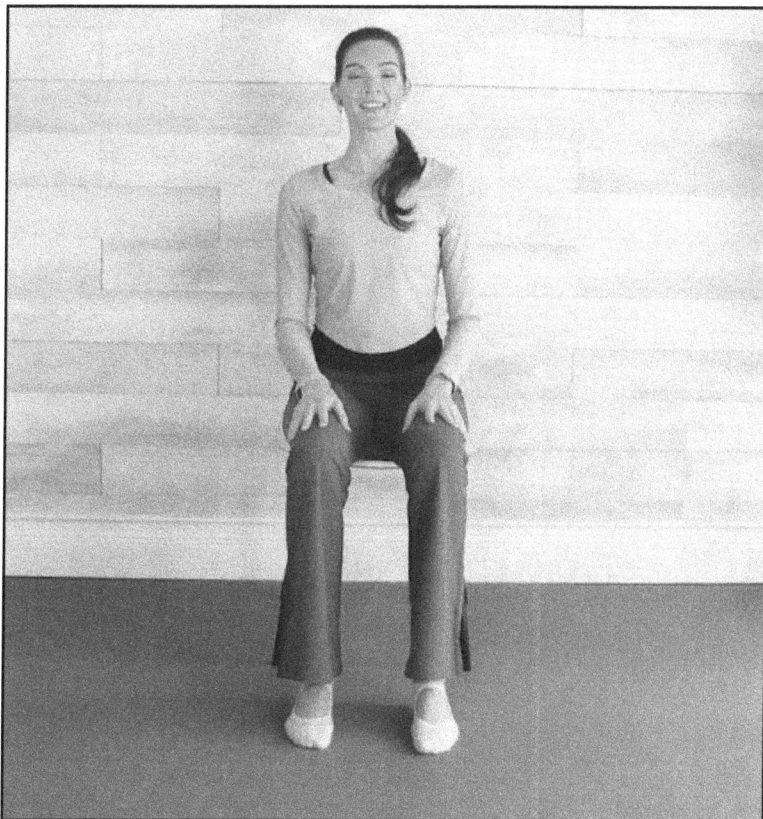

Gently scan your body — notice your shoulders,   jaw, back, and hands.

Ask: "Where am I holding tension?"

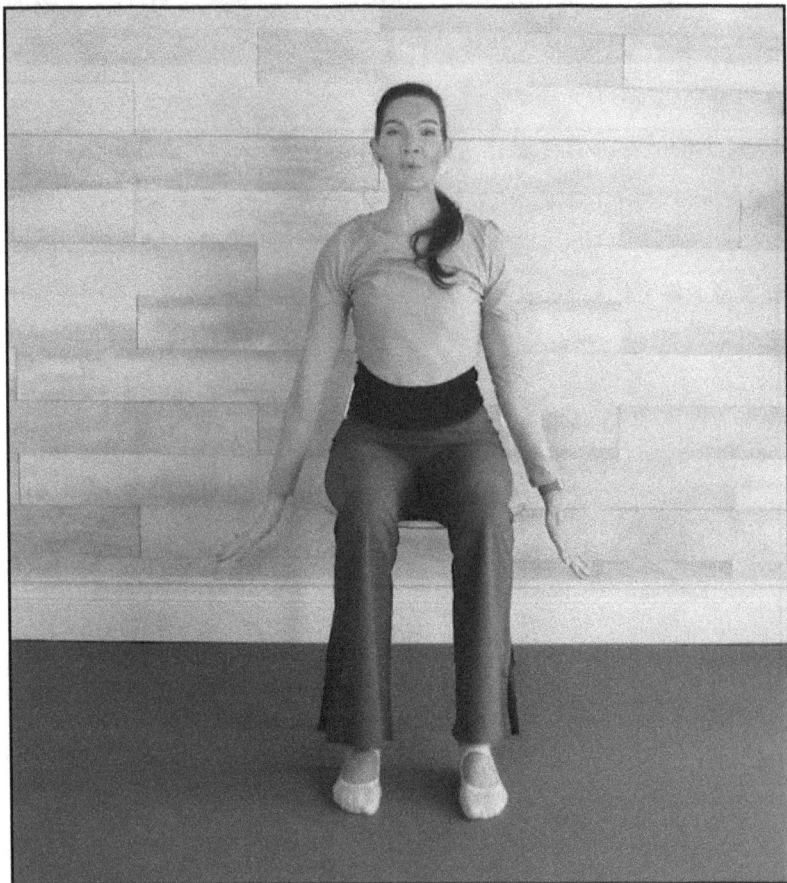

- Release what you can:

- Gently move the area of your body where you feel tension.

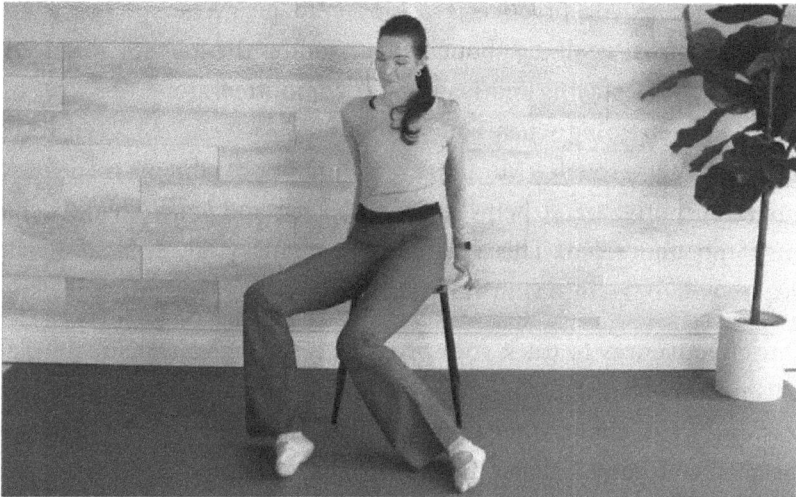

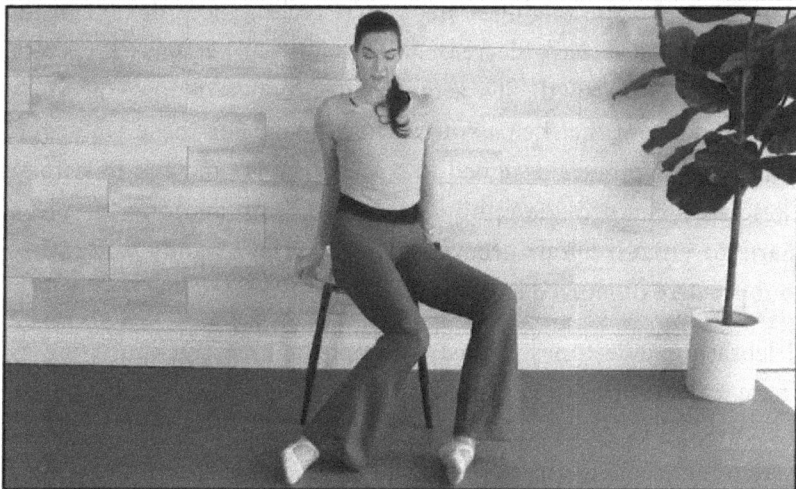

6.3 TRACKING PROGRESS AND CELEBRATING MILESTONES

Imagine climbing a mountain. Each step forward brings you closer to the peak, no matter how small. This is what tracking progress in somatic exercises feels like. It's about recognizing the small victories that happen as you practice. Tracking your progress isn't just about reaching a final goal; it's about understanding the journey that leads to it. It's about staying motivated and committed along the way. It's easier to keep going when you see how far you've come, even when the path gets tough. Monitoring your improvements can be a powerful motivator. It helps you see the big and small changes that might go unnoticed. This awareness can fuel your dedication and inspire you to tap into your full potential.

One effective way to track your progress is through a somatic journal. This notebook can be where you jot down your experiences after each session. Write about what exercises you did, how you felt, and any insights you gained. Over time, you'll start to notice patterns and improvements. You might see that you're feeling more flexible or that your stress levels have decreased. This journal becomes a personal record of your growth. It's a tangible reminder of how far you've come and a tool that helps you set new goals. For those who prefer digital tools, apps are designed to track practice time and milestones. These apps can provide reminders, log sessions, and offer graphs or charts to visualize your progress. They can be a handy way to keep your practice organized and on track.

Celebrating milestones is just as important as tracking progress. These celebrations don't need to be grand. What's important is acknowledging your achievements. Consider creating a reward system for reaching goals. This could be as simple as treating yourself to a favorite activity or enjoying a special meal. Rewards can serve as a positive reinforcement, encouraging continued effort. Sharing successes with a supportive community can also be rewarding. Whether it's family, friends, or an online group, sharing your achievements can provide encouragement and motivation. It creates a sense of connection and shared joy, making the journey feel less lonely and more meaningful.

Reflection on progress is a crucial part of this process. Taking the time to reflect on your achievements reinforces your motivation and commitment to your goals. Reflective entries in your practice journal can be helpful in this regard. Write about how you've grown and what you've learned. Consider what challenges you've overcome and how you've handled setbacks. This reflection can deepen your understanding of your practice. It highlights your strengths and areas for improvement, providing a clearer picture of where you stand. By recognizing your achievements, you build a sense of pride and accomplishment. This, in turn, strengthens your resolve to continue.

Interactive Element: Progress Reflection Prompt

- **Weekly Reflection**: At the end of each week, take a moment to note down any achievements or insights from your practice. What are you proud of? What did you learn? What would you like to focus on next week?

Tracking progress and celebrating milestones in somatic practice is a powerful way to stay motivated and engaged. It transforms the process from a series of exercises into a meaningful and rewarding personal experience. By acknowledging your efforts and reflecting on your growth, you foster a deeper connection with yourself and your practice. This connection enhances your somatic journey and enriches your life, encouraging continued exploration and discovery.

6.4 PERSONALIZING YOUR SOMATIC PRACTICE

When it comes to somatic exercises, one size does not fit all. Personalizing your routine is key to unlocking its full potential. Tailoring exercises to your needs can make all the difference. Why does this matter? The answer is simple: personal preferences can make or break your practice. Choosing exercises that align with your interests and abilities increases your likelihood of sticking with them. This consistency leads to better results and a more enjoyable experience. Focusing on what works for you makes the practice more effective and fulfilling.

Customizing your somatic exercises begins with understanding your goals and abilities. Modifications are crucial for specific physical conditions, such as back pain or joint issues. For instance, if bending forward causes discomfort, try a gentler stretch or use props for support. This adaptation ensures that your practice remains safe and beneficial. It's also essential to choose focus areas based on personal interests. If you're drawn to improving flexibility, prioritize exercises that stretch and lengthen muscles. If stress relief is your goal, incorporate calming breathwork and gentle movements to achieve it. Selecting exercises that resonate with you makes your practice more meaningful and rewarding.

Experimentation plays a vital role in finding what works best for you. Trying different approaches can help you discover your ideal practice. Experiment with various exercise styles and techniques to determine what feels most comfortable for you. You might explore a mix of yoga-inspired movements, breathwork, or dance-like flows. Each style offers unique benefits, and experimenting allows you to find the perfect combination that suits you. As your needs change, adapt your routines accordingly. Life is dynamic, and so should your practice be. If you find a specific exercise no longer serves you, don't hesitate to adjust it or try something new. This flexibility ensures your practice evolves with you, keeping it fresh and engaging.

The advantages of a personalized somatic practice are numerous. When you tailor exercises to your needs, you increase engagement and enjoyment. This leads to greater satisfaction and more consistent practice. You may look forward to your sessions, eager to explore new movements and sensations. This enthusiasm translates into better results, both physically and emotionally. Personal stories highlight the success of customized routines. Take Jane, for example, who tailored her practice to focus on stress relief. She found a sense of calm and balance in her daily life by incorporating breathwork and gentle stretches into her routine. Similarly, Tom, who struggled with flexibility, modified his routine to prioritize stretching. Over time, he noticed significant improvements in his range of motion and overall comfort. These stories demonstrate how personalization can lead to transformative outcomes.

Embracing a personalized approach empowers you to take ownership of your practice. It encourages self-discovery and self-care, fostering a deeper connection with your body. You create a practice that supports your well-being by listening to your needs and preferences. This approach enhances your physical health and nurtures your emotional and mental well-being. As you continue to explore and adapt your practice, you'll uncover new insights about yourself and your body's capabilities. This journey of personalization is not just about the exercises themselves. It's about cultivating a practice that aligns with your values and goals, one that evolves in tandem with you.

The next chapter will delve into advanced techniques to further enhance your somatic practice. These methods will build upon your established foundations, offering new ways to deepen your connection with your body and mind.

CHAPTER 7

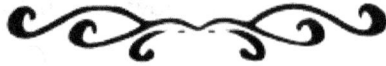

OVERCOMING COMMON CHALLENGES AND MAINTAINING MOTIVATION

I magine you're tending a garden. You water it daily, hoping to see vibrant blooms. But after weeks, the plants seem to remain unchanged. You feel frustration creeping in. This scenario mirrors the experience of hitting a plateau in your somatic practice. Everything feels stagnant. Plateaus can be disheartening, leaving you questioning the value of your efforts. They often manifest as a lack of noticeable progress in flexibility or strength. You might find your enthusiasm waning, turning each session into a chore rather than a joy. Recognizing these signs is the first step in addressing them.

Plateaus occur for various reasons. Repetitive routines can lead to boredom, making sessions feel monotonous and unengaging. When you follow the same set of exercises repeatedly, your body becomes accustomed to them. This adaptation causes progress to level out. Your muscles become accustomed to the movements, reducing the stimulus required for growth. Insufficient challenge or variety can also contribute to this issue. Without introducing new elements or increasing difficulty, your practice may feel stagnant. These factors can diminish motivation, making it harder to stay engaged. Understanding these causes provides clarity and helps you identify areas for change.

To overcome plateaus, consider introducing new exercises or techniques to challenge your progress. This doesn't mean abandoning your routine entirely but incorporating fresh elements. Trying different activities can engage various muscle groups, reigniting interest and challenge. For example, if you've focused on seated stretches, incorporate standing poses to engage other parts of your body. Increasing the intensity or duration can also be helpful. Gradually extending the length of your sessions or adding additional reps can stimulate growth. These changes can rekindle your enthusiasm and breathe new life into your practice.

It's crucial to approach plateaus with patience and persistence. They are a natural part of any practice and can be overcome with time and effort. Trust the process and remain committed to your goals. Even if it feels repetitive, each session contributes to your long-term progress. Embrace the idea that growth is not always linear. Some periods may seem stagnant, but they often precede breakthroughs. Remember the garden analogy: while growth might not be visible immediately, it doesn't mean it's not happening beneath the surface.

Interactive Element: Reflection Journal

Consider keeping a journal to reflect on your experiences and record your thoughts. After each session, jot down your observations. Note any changes in how your body feels or shifts in your mindset. Reflect on moments of frustration and breakthroughs. This practice can provide insights into your progress and highlight areas for improvement. It also serves as a reminder of how far you've come, reinforcing your commitment and resilience.

By embracing these strategies, you can transform your approach to somatic exercises. They encourage you to challenge yourself and explore new possibilities. You can navigate plateaus and continue your journey toward enhanced well-being with patience and persistence.

Maintaining high motivation is crucial for success in somatic practice. Motivation acts like the fuel that keeps your practice going. It helps you show up daily, even when you're tired or busy. When motivation is strong, it encourages consistency. Consistency is what turns practice into a habit. Over time, these habits lead to real progress. You see changes in how you move and feel, which boosts your confidence and keeps you engaged. Without motivation, it's easy to skip sessions or lose interest in them. That's why finding ways to stay motivated is key. It ensures you keep moving forward, even when challenges arise.

One way to stay motivated is by setting short-term, achievable goals. These goals give you something to aim for. They break down your larger objectives into smaller, more manageable steps. For example, instead of focusing on perfecting a complex movement, start with a simpler one. Celebrate when you achieve it. These small wins add up, building your confidence and momentum. Another way to stay motivated is by using motivational quotes or affirmations. Place them where you can see them often, like on your mirror or desk. These reminders can inspire you, especially when you're feeling low. They remind you of why you started and what you're working toward.

Creating a vision board can also boost motivation. A vision board is a collection of images and words that reflect your goals and dreams. It serves as a visual reminder of where you want to go. Fill it with inspiring pictures, quotes that move you, and goals that excite you. Place it somewhere you'll see every day. Glancing at it can reignite your passion and focus, keeping your motivation alive. It's a powerful tool that helps you visualize your future and stay connected to your aspirations.

Celebrating small victories plays a significant role in maintaining motivation. Recognizing and celebrating achievements, no matter how small, reinforces positive behavior—plan mini-rewards for reaching milestones. Enjoy a favorite treat, take a relaxing bath, or spend time doing something you love. These rewards acknowledge your hard work and dedication. They make the journey enjoyable and give you something to look forward to. Celebrating successes keeps the process positive, encouraging you to strive for more.

Personal stories and testimonials can provide inspiration and reassurance. Hearing how others have stayed motivated can offer fresh perspectives and ideas. Take, for example, Sarah, who struggled to maintain her practice during a busy work season. She began setting small goals, such as practicing for ten minutes a day. Over time, she noticed her motivation returning. She began to feel the benefits of her practice, which encouraged her to keep going. Then there's Tom, who felt stuck after months of practice. He created a vision board that served as a reminder of his long-term goals. This simple act reignited his passion and helped him stay committed to his goals. These stories show that everyone faces challenges, but with the right tools, you can overcome them.

Motivation is not a constant state. It can ebb and flow. But by implementing these strategies, you can keep it alive and thriving. Setting goals, using affirmations, creating vision boards, and celebrating victories all contribute to a motivated mindset. These tools provide the support you need to stay on track and achieve your goals. They remind you of the progress you've made and the potential that lies ahead. With motivation as your ally, you can continue to grow and thrive in your somatic practice.

7.2 DEALING WITH SELF-DOUBT AND FEAR OF FAILURE

Self-doubt often creeps into somatic practice, casting shadows on your progress. It can arise from comparing yourself to others. You may see someone who seems more flexible or stronger and feels inadequate. These comparisons can undermine confidence, leading you to question your abilities. Another source of self-doubt comes from setting unrealistic expectations. You might expect rapid results or flawless execution, forgetting that growth takes time and practice. When reality doesn't match these high standards, doubt can become overwhelming. These feelings can hold you back, making it hard to see the progress you've already made.

To combat self-doubt and fear, practice self-compassion and kindness. Treat yourself as you would a close friend in need of support. Acknowledge your efforts and celebrate your small victories. When negative thoughts arise, try reframing them into positive affirmations. Instead of thinking, "I'll never get this right," tell yourself, "I'm improving with each practice." This shift in mindset can transform doubt into encouragement. Visualization exercises can also help. Picture yourself succeeding in your practice. Imagine each movement flowing smoothly and feel the confidence it brings. These mental rehearsals can build belief in your abilities and boost your self-esteem.

Adopting a growth mindset is also a powerful way to tackle self-doubt. This perspective views challenges as opportunities for learning rather than threats. When you encounter difficulties, view them as opportunities for growth. Every mistake becomes a lesson, not a failure. This mindset fosters resilience, allowing you to bounce back from setbacks with renewed determination. It encourages you to embrace the learning process, knowing that each step, no matter how small, contributes to your development. By focusing on growth rather than perfection, you create a more positive and supportive environment for yourself.

Support systems play a crucial role in overcoming self-doubt. A strong network of friends, mentors, or coaches can provide encouragement and reassurance. They offer different perspectives, helping you see your strengths and potential. Seek guidance from those who understand your struggles and can offer practical advice. A mentor or coach can help you navigate challenges, providing insights and strategies to overcome obstacles. Their support can bolster your confidence, reminding you you're not alone. Sharing your experiences with others also creates a sense of community, where you can learn from each other's journeys and celebrate successes together.

Incorporating these strategies into your practice can transform self-doubt into self-assurance. By practicing self-compassion and kindness, you nurture a positive relationship with yourself. Reframing negative thoughts and utilizing visualization exercises helps build confidence and resilience. Adopting a growth mindset encourages you to see challenges as opportunities for learning and growth. Surrounding yourself with a supportive network offers encouragement and guidance. These tools help you navigate the ups and downs of somatic practice with grace and perseverance. You learn to trust in your abilities and embrace the process, knowing that each step forward brings you closer to your goals.

7.3 MAINTAINING CONSISTENCY IN YOUR PRACTICE

Maintaining consistency in your practice is like building a sturdy bridge. Every small, regular effort adds strength. With each plank you lay, the path becomes more secure. Regular practice yields steady progress, helping you turn your goals into reality. As you practice regularly, your body learns and adapts to the movements you perform. Repeated actions form habits, and these habits shape your skills. This is how you achieve lasting results. When you show up consistently, you give yourself the chance to improve. Your body grows more substantial and more flexible. Your mind becomes more focused and calm. Over time, these small steps forward add up to significant changes.

Building a consistent routine starts with setting specific times for practice. Treat this time as an essential appointment with yourself. Make it a priority first thing in the morning or just before bed. Select a time that suits your daily schedule. Once you decide, stick to it as much as you can. This regularity helps make practice a natural part of your day. Habit-tracking tools or apps can help. These tools remind you of your practice time. They also let you see your progress at a glance. Watching your streak grow can motivate you to keep going. It becomes a visual reminder of your commitment and effort.

Accountability plays a key role in maintaining consistency. When someone else is counting on you, showing up is more manageable. Find a practice partner or accountability buddy. This person can join your sessions or check in with you. Knowing that a friend is there can push you to keep your commitment. If finding a partner isn't possible, consider joining online somatic groups. These communities often have shared goals. They provide support and encouragement. Being part of a group adds a social element to your practice. It makes the experience more enjoyable and less lonely. You can share tips, celebrate successes, and support each other through challenges.

Life often throws curveballs that disrupt routines. A busy week at work or sudden travel plans can make it hard to keep up with practice. When this happens, don't be too hard on yourself. Instead, focus on getting back on track. If you miss a session, don't give up. Resume your practice as soon as you can. A break doesn't erase your progress. It's just a pause. Adjust your schedule to fit your current circumstances. If you can't manage an entire session, try a shorter one. Flexibility is key. It allows you to adapt without losing momentum.

When schedules change, creativity can be a valuable asset. If you find yourself with a spare moment, use it. A few minutes of focused breathing or a quick stretch can keep your practice alive. These small actions remind your body and mind of what you've been working on. They maintain the connection between sessions. Consistency isn't about perfection. It's about making practice a regular part of your life. Even when life gets busy, these small efforts count. They support your progress and keep you moving forward.

As you work to maintain consistency, remember why you started. Recall the benefits you've felt and the goals you set. Let them guide your actions. Consistency helps you build the bridge to where you want to go. Each step you take strengthens it. It creates a reliable and strong path, leading you toward the changes you seek.

○→ Sit on a mat.

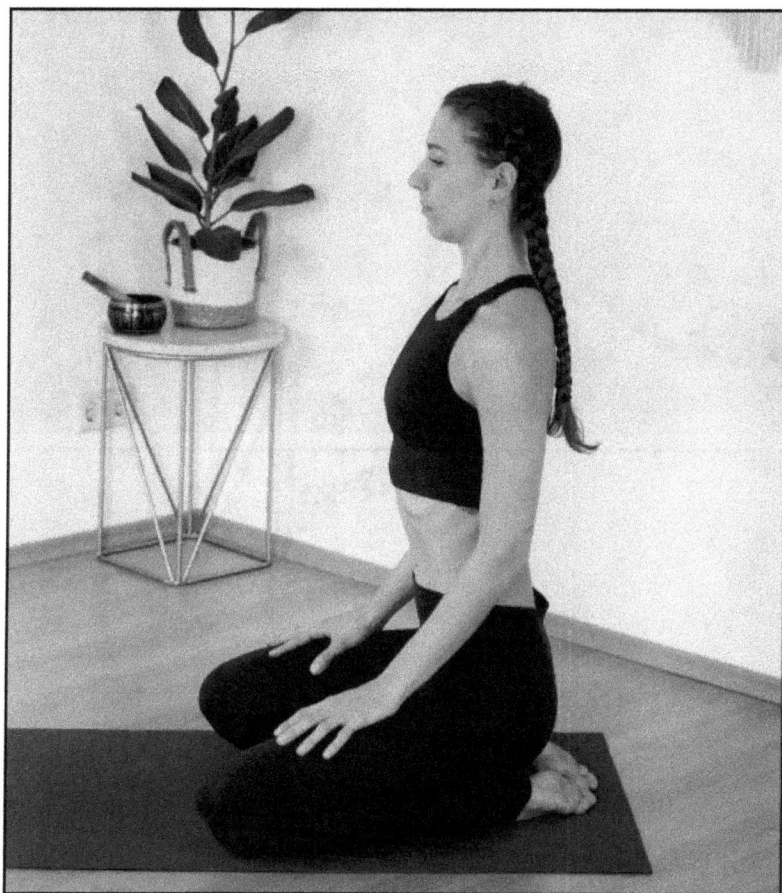

- Kneel and fold forward, arms stretched ahead or by sides.

- Rest forehead down, breathe deeply for 3-4 breaths.

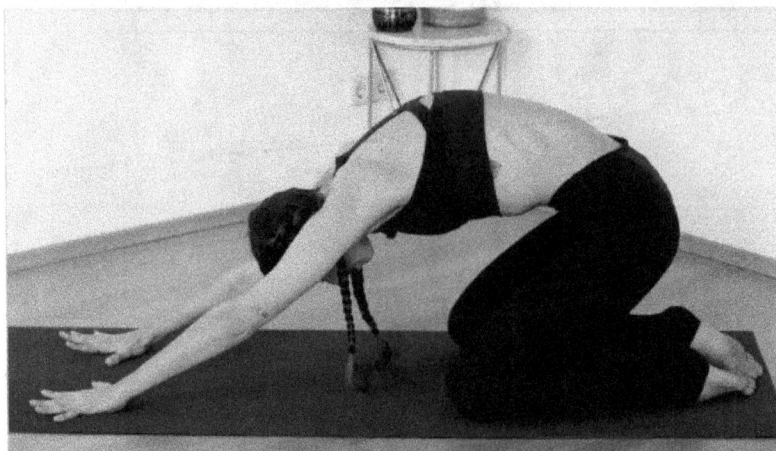

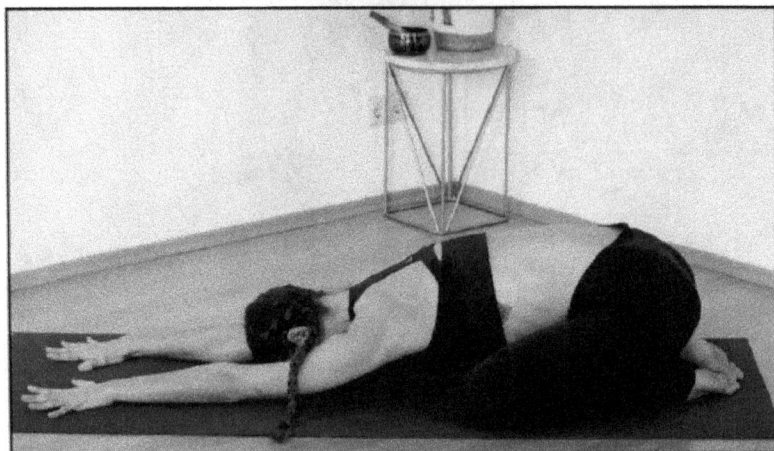

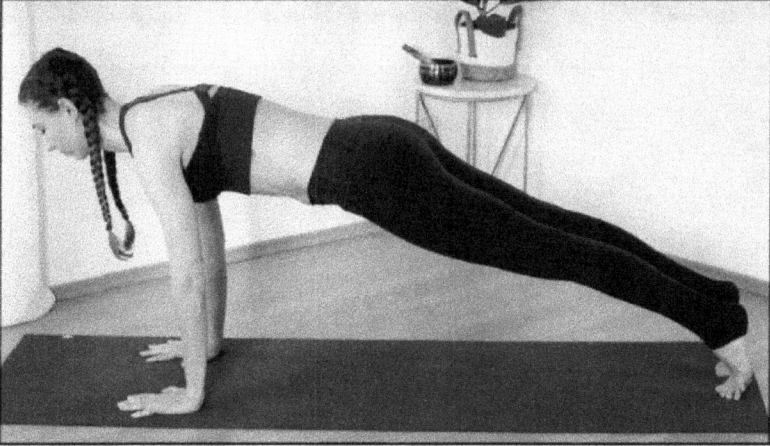

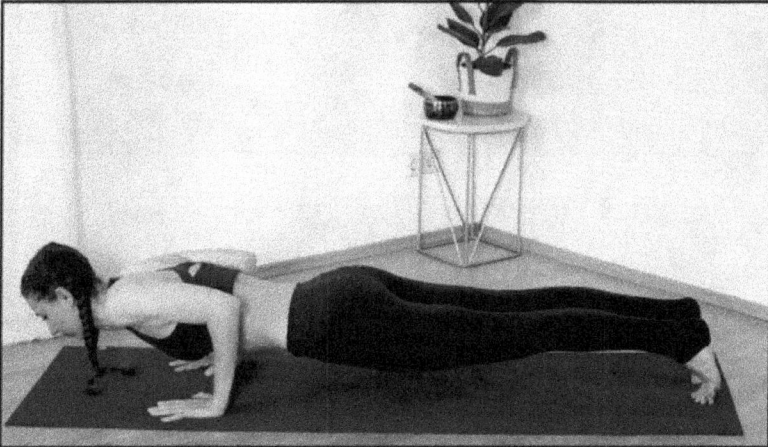

123

- From plank, lower hips toward the floor, straighten arms.

- Open the chest, lift through the heart, and hold for 2-3 breaths.

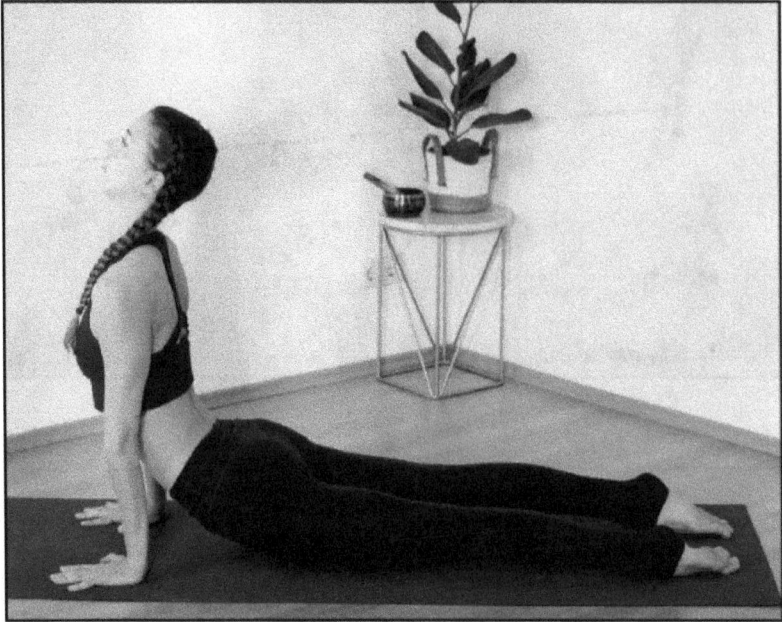

- Lift hips up and back into an inverted "V."

- Press heels gently toward the ground, lengthen the spine.

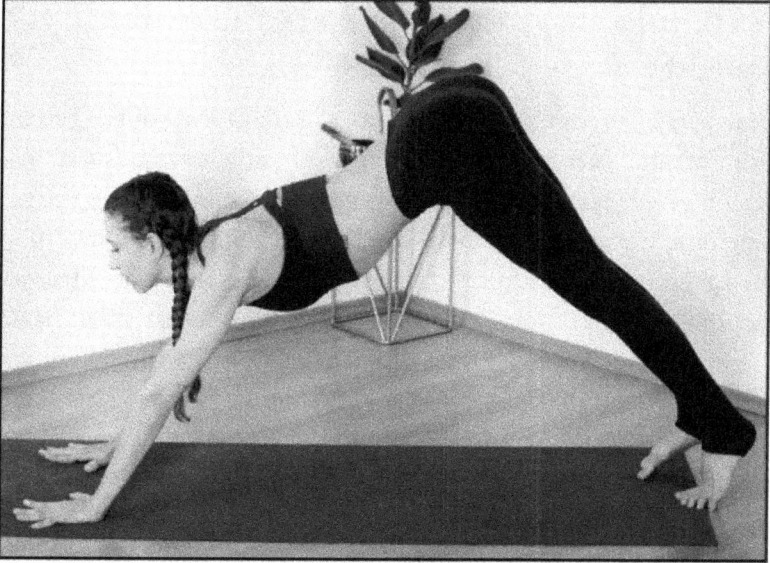

Hold for 3-5 breaths before resting.

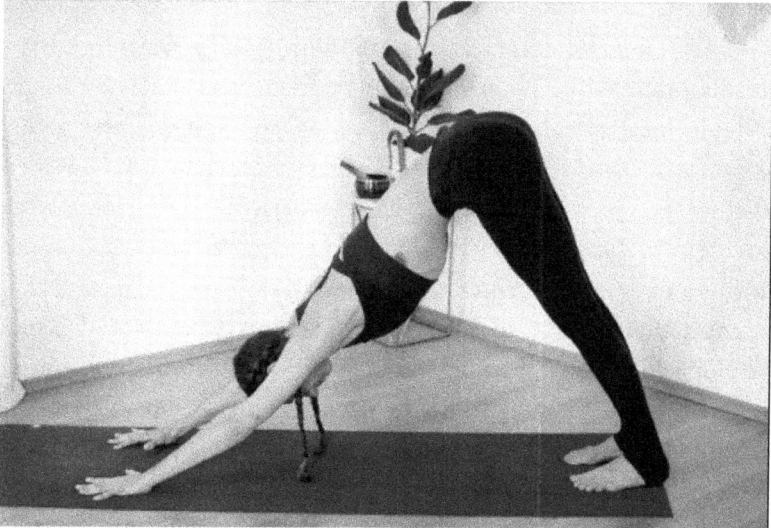

7.4 FINDING SUPPORT AND BUILDING A SOMATIC COMMUNITY

Being part of a supportive community can transform your experience with somatic exercises. Connecting with others who share your passion gives you a sense of belonging. This feeling of being part of something bigger can motivate you to keep going, even when things get tough. A community offers encouragement that lifts you, providing the push you need to continue. It's not just about having people around you; it's about sharing a journey with others who understand your challenges and share in your victories. This shared experience can make your practice more fulfilling and enjoyable. You also gain access to a wealth of knowledge and different perspectives. As you interact with others, you learn new techniques and insights. These exchanges can deepen your understanding and enhance your practice. Sharing experiences with peers can inspire you to try new approaches and refine your skills. They provide a platform for growth that extends beyond solitary practice.

Building a somatic community starts with finding ways to connect with like-minded individuals. One way to achieve this is by participating in local somatic exercise classes or workshops. These gatherings offer a space to connect with others who share your interests. Whether you're a beginner or have experience, these classes can provide new insights and techniques to explore. You might find a class at a community center, gym, or wellness studio. These settings foster an environment of learning and support where you can practice alongside others. If in-person meetings aren't an option, consider participating in online forums or social media groups. These platforms offer a virtual space for connecting with people from all over the world. They allow you to share experiences, ask questions, and provide support. You can join groups that focus on specific aspects of somatic exercises, connecting with others who share similar goals and interests.

Sharing knowledge and experiences is a powerful way to engage with your community. When you contribute your insights, you enrich the collective understanding. Hosting or attending virtual practice meetups can be an excellent way to connect with others and share your knowledge. These gatherings provide a platform for sharing techniques and learning from one another. You can discuss challenges, celebrate successes, and offer support. They create a sense of camaraderie and collaboration, enhancing your practice. Sharing personal stories and insights with peers can also be a valuable experience. You invite others to do the same when you open up about your experiences. These exchanges build trust and deepen connections. They remind you that you're not alone in your practice, fostering a sense of solidarity and camaraderie.

For many, community involvement has had a profound impact on their practice. Consider Jane, who attended a local workshop and met others with similar interests. She found new friends who kept her motivated and inspired. Their shared practice sessions became a highlight of her week. Another example is Tom, who joined an online group dedicated to somatic exercises. The support and encouragement he received helped him overcome challenges. He felt a renewed sense of purpose and excitement for his practice. These testimonials highlight how community involvement can enhance motivation and success. When you find your tribe, you gain a support system that encourages growth and exploration.

As you reflect on the possibilities of building a somatic community, consider how these connections can enrich your practice and enhance your overall well-being. They provide a space for learning, sharing, and growth. By engaging with others, you expand your horizons and gain new insights. This support can make your practice more rewarding and meaningful. Embrace the opportunities to connect and learn from those around you. Together, you can create a community that uplifts and inspires, supporting each other in the pursuit of well-being.

Chapter 7 explored overcoming challenges like plateaus, motivation, and self-doubt. Building a supportive community enhances your practice. Next, we'll delve into advanced emotional and physical healing techniques, offering more profound insights into somatic exercises.

Micro-Practice Consistency Routine

Cat-Cow Stretch

- Start on hands and knees.

- Exhale, round your spine upward, tuck chin toward chest.

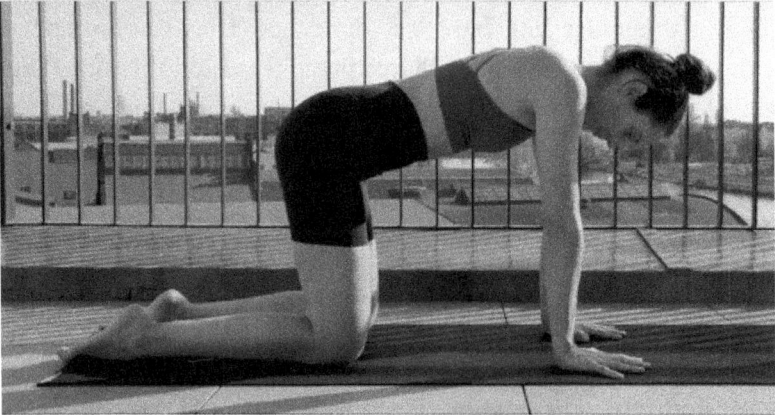

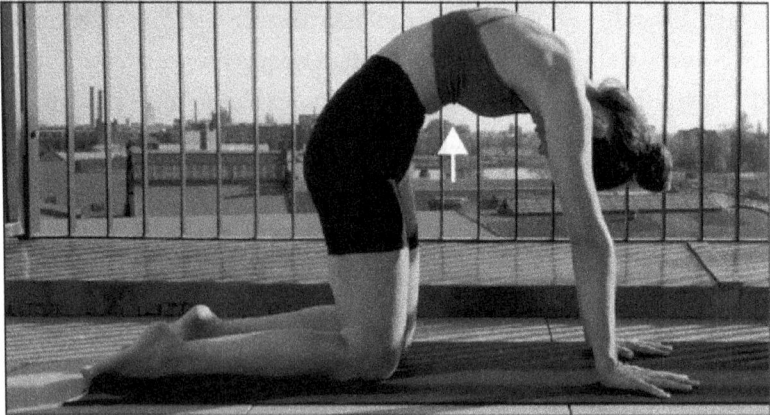

Inhale, arch your spine, lift chest and tailbone gently upward.

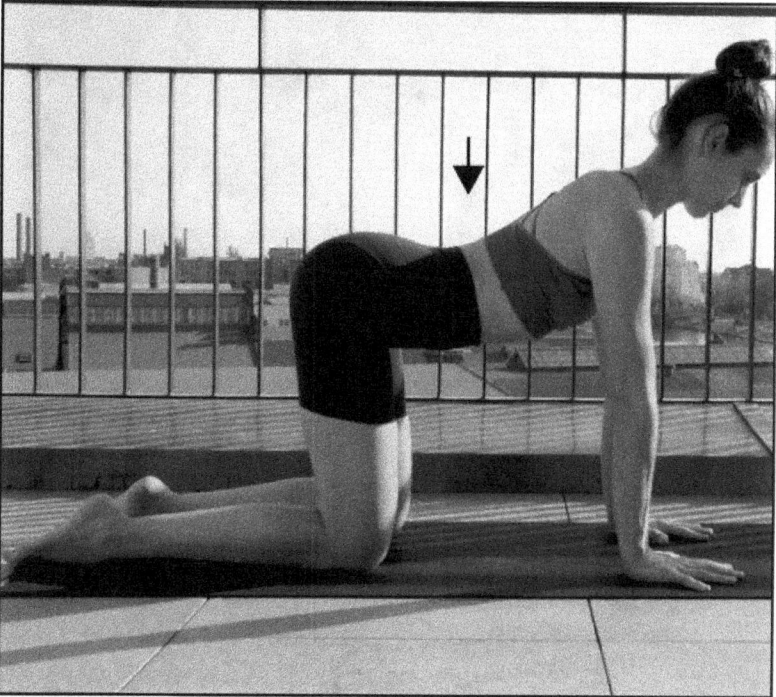

Move slowly between Cat and Cow for 3-5 breaths.

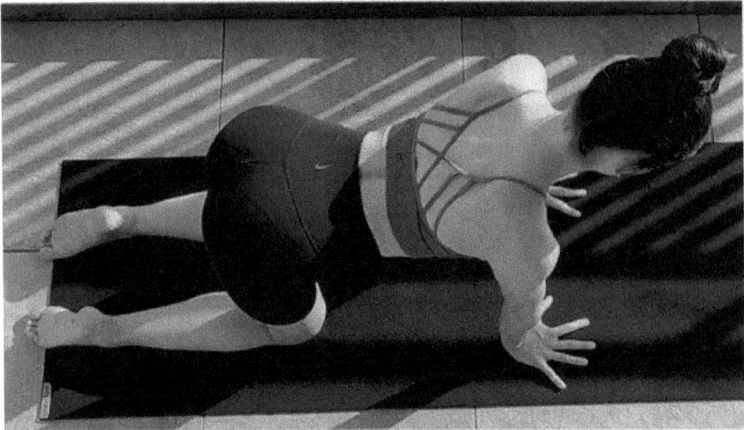

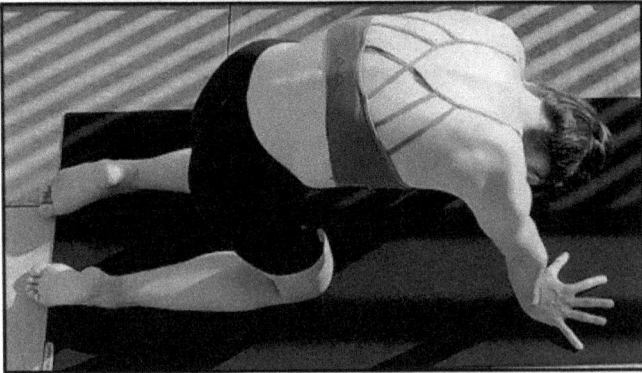

Let this short practice build into a natural daily habit.

CHAPTER 8

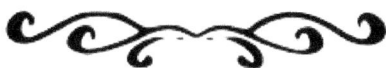

ADVANCED TECHNIQUES FOR EMOTIONAL AND PHYSICAL HEALING

I magine standing at the edge of a vast, open field. The air is clear, and a gentle breeze caresses your skin. This moment of stillness and clarity reflects the potential of advanced breathwork. It offers a pathway to emotional release and healing. Breathwork is not just about breathing; it's about connecting deeply with your emotions. It allows you to explore your inner world with intention and awareness. Techniques such as holotropic breathing and rebirthing breathwork are potent tools on this journey. They guide you toward a state of openness where healing can take root.

Holotropic breathing involves controlled, quickened breaths that lead you into an altered state of consciousness. This practice was developed by psychiatrists Stanislav and Christina Grof in the 1970s. They aimed to mimic the effects of psychedelics without drugs, offering a safe way to explore consciousness. You breathe rapidly and evenly during a session, often accompanied by rhythmic music. This process can bring hidden emotions to the surface, allowing you to confront and release them. It's an opportunity to delve into your mind and emotions, fostering personal growth and self-awareness.

Rebirthing breathwork is another technique that facilitates emotional release. It focuses on circular breathing without pauses between breaths. The continuous flow of air helps you access repressed emotions and memories. You may feel that old wounds resurface as you breathe, but this is a natural part of the healing process. Acknowledging and releasing these emotions creates space for new insights and clarity. Rebirthing breathwork is a gentle yet profound way to explore your emotional landscape. It connects you to your breath and body, fostering a sense of wholeness and peace.

When practicing advanced breathwork, safety is paramount. Working with a trained facilitator who can guide you through the process is best. They ensure you remain grounded and safe as you explore deeper emotional states. Sessions usually last 60 to 90 minutes in a quiet, comfortable environment. It's essential to listen to your body and take breaks if needed. Avoid practicing these techniques if you have certain medical conditions, like cardiovascular issues or severe mental illness. The presence of a facilitator helps maintain a safe and supportive space, allowing you to focus on your breath and emotions.

The emotional benefits of advanced breathwork are significant. Many people experience breakthroughs that lead to healing and transformation. For example, one person who struggled with anxiety found relief through holotropic breathing. During a session, they confronted and released old fears, feeling lighter and more at peace afterward. Another individual used rebirthing breathwork to process grief. By facing their emotions head-on, they found closure and healing. These stories demonstrate the transformative power of breathwork in fostering emotional clarity and personal growth. It's a unique journey that helps you connect with yourself more deeply.

To integrate breathwork into your routine, create a dedicated space for practice. Find a quiet corner in your home where you can breathe freely without distractions. Consider using cushions or a yoga mat for comfort. You can also combine breathwork with other somatic exercises for enhanced effects. For instance, begin your session with a body scan to ground yourself, then transition into breathwork. This combination deepens your connection to your body and emotions. It offers a holistic approach to healing that nurtures both mind and body. Regular practice reinforces the benefits, helping you navigate life's challenges more easily.

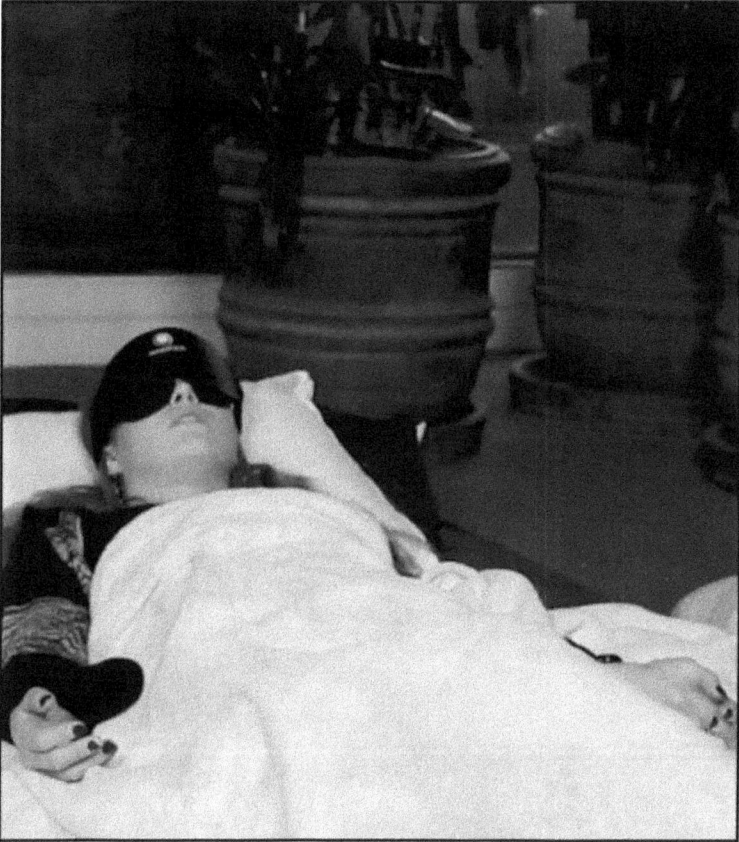

- Lie on your back or sit supported in a quiet space.

- Close your eyes or use a sleep masks and take 2-3 grounding breaths. Set an intention (e.g., "gentle release" or "trust").

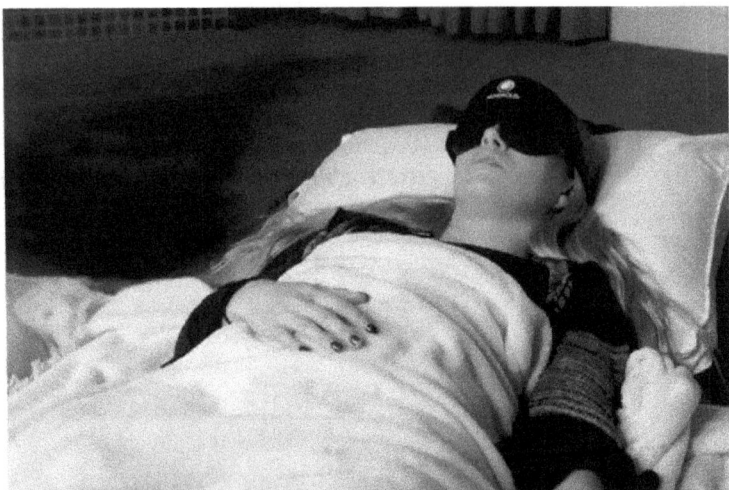

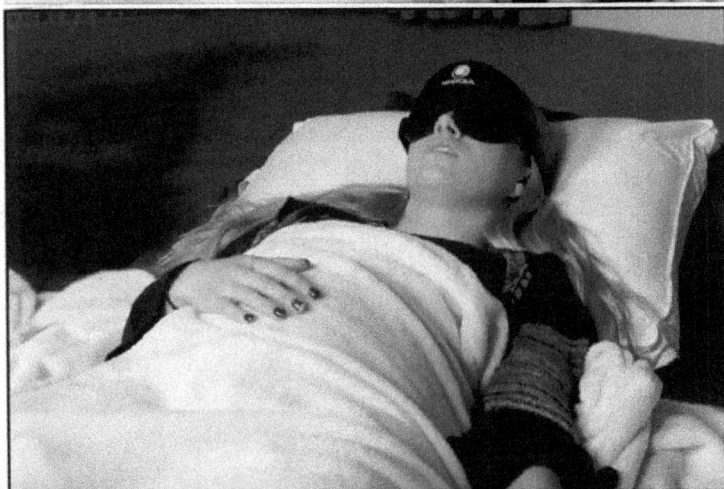

- Inhale through your mouth in a steady, full breath.
- Exhale immediately and fully through your mouth — without pausing at the top or bottom.
- Keep the rhythm continuous: in, out, in, out.

Keep the pace moderate. If intensity builds, return to nose breathing or pause for a few breaths.

Observe sensations without judgment.

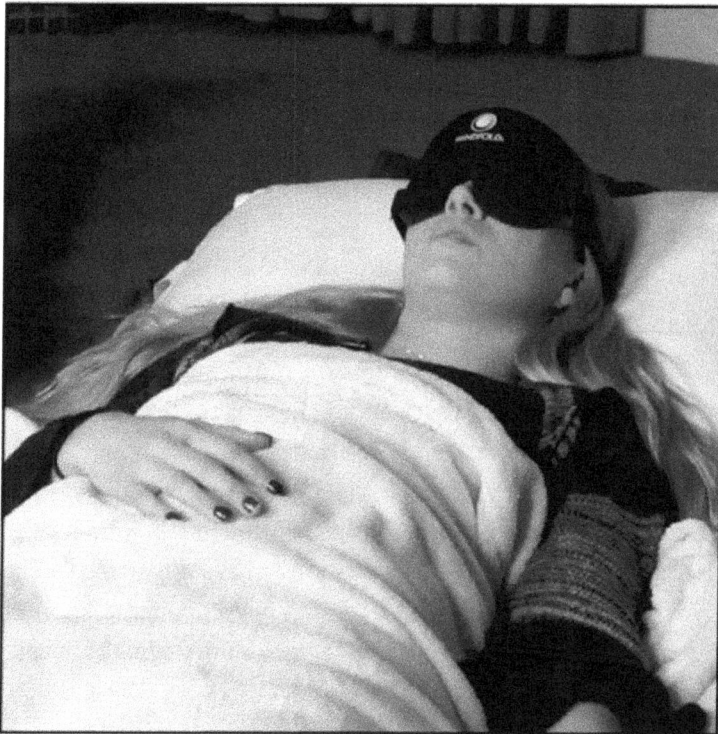

Continue for 1-3 minutes, then return to normal breathing and rest.

8.1 EXPLORING INTUITIVE MOVEMENT FOR DEEPER CONNECTION

Imagine moving in a way that feels completely natural and unplanned. This is intuitive movement, where your body leads without strict rules or expectations. It helps you connect your mind and body, guiding you to move based on how you feel rather than how you think you should move. Intuition plays a key role here. It allows you to express yourself physically in a way that feels right at that moment. This movement can reveal emotional truths, bringing hidden feelings to the surface. When you let your body move freely, you might discover emotions you didn't know existed. This process can enlighten you, offering insights into your feelings and their underlying causes.

There are many ways to explore intuitive movement. Free-form dance sessions are a great start. Put on music you love and let your body respond to it. Don't worry about steps or rhythm. Focus on how the music makes you feel and let that guide your movement. You might sway, twirl, or even stomp. The goal is to move in a way that feels good and true to you. Another option is to join movement improvisation workshops. These sessions provide a space to explore different ways of moving with others. They encourage spontaneity and creativity, helping you break away from rigid patterns and discover new possibilities.

Embracing intuitive movement can transform your mind and body. It enhances self-awareness, enabling you to understand your body and emotions more effectively. This awareness can lead to emotional release, helping you release tension and stress. As you move intuitively, you'll also find that your creativity blossoms. The freedom to explore new movements encourages you to express yourself uniquely. This self-expression can be incredibly empowering, boosting your confidence and self-esteem. It connects you to your body on a deeper level, enhancing your overall well-being and resilience.

However, not everyone finds it easy to start with intuitive movement. You might feel self-conscious or worry about being judged. It's normal to feel this way at first. One strategy to overcome this is to practice in a private, comfortable setting. This could be your living room, a quiet park, or any other space where you feel at ease. Without the pressure of an audience, you can focus on your experience and how it feels. Another approach is to let go of judgment. Remind yourself that there is no right or wrong way to move. Embrace spontaneity and allow your body to take the lead. You might be surprised by how liberating this can be.

Somatic Experiencing

Somatic Yin Yoga Flow

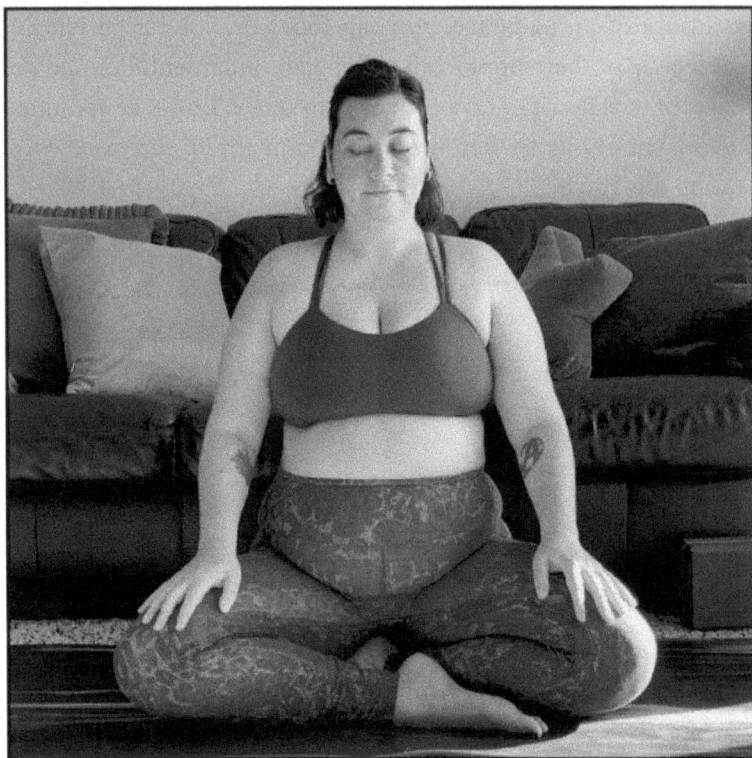

- Sit or lie down comfortably.

- Pause and notice one area of your body — it can be tense, calm, or neutral.

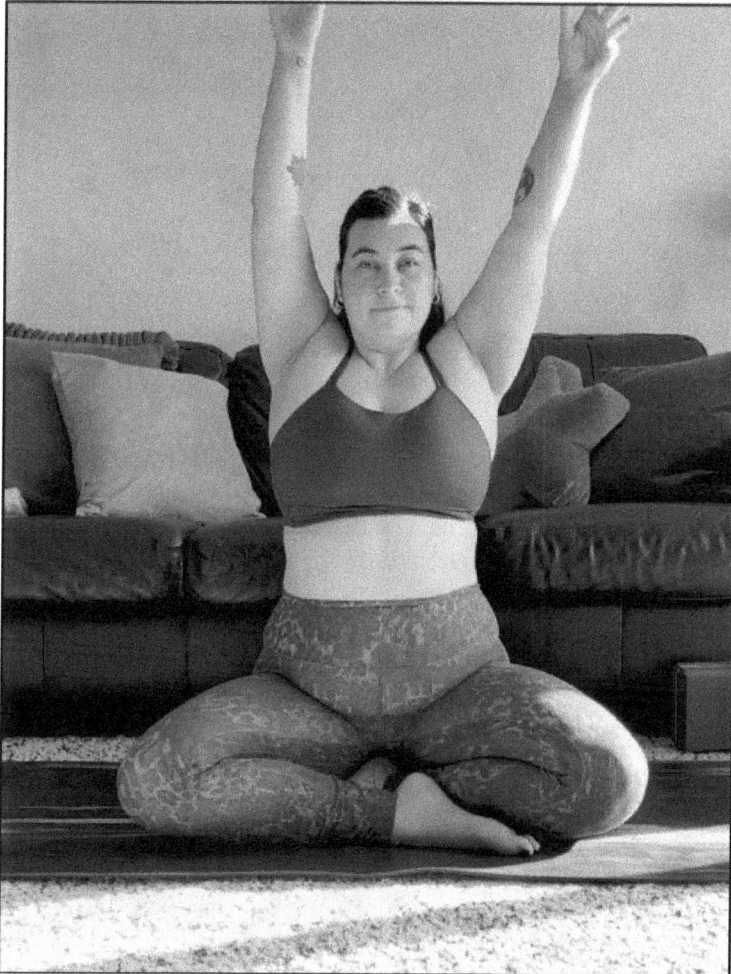

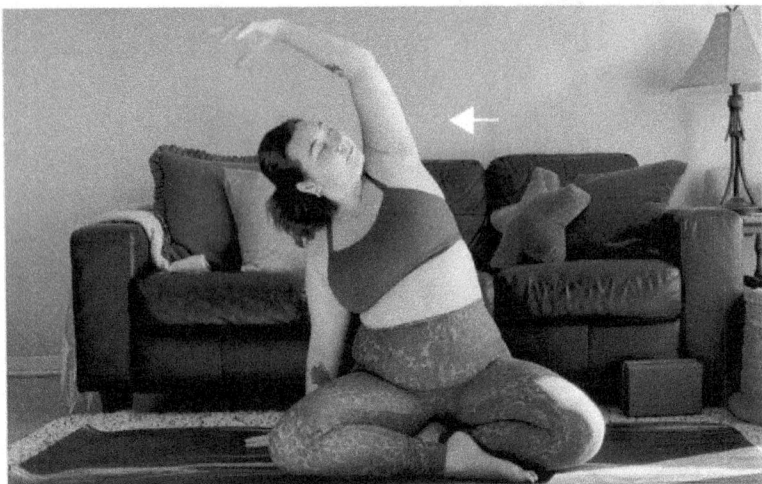

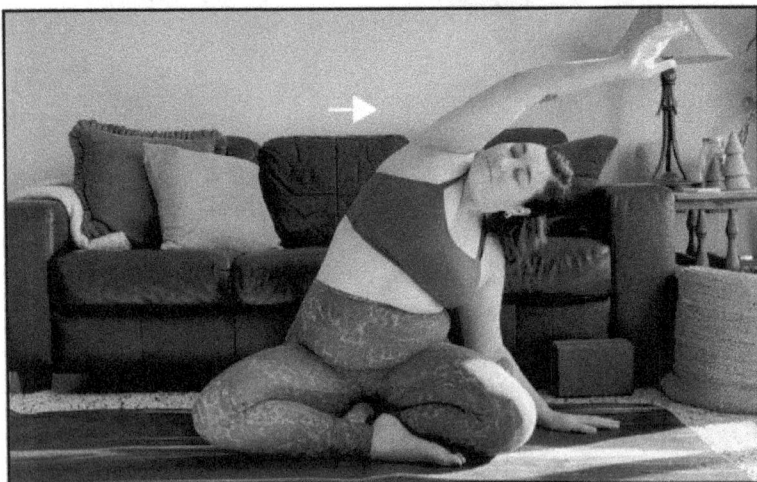

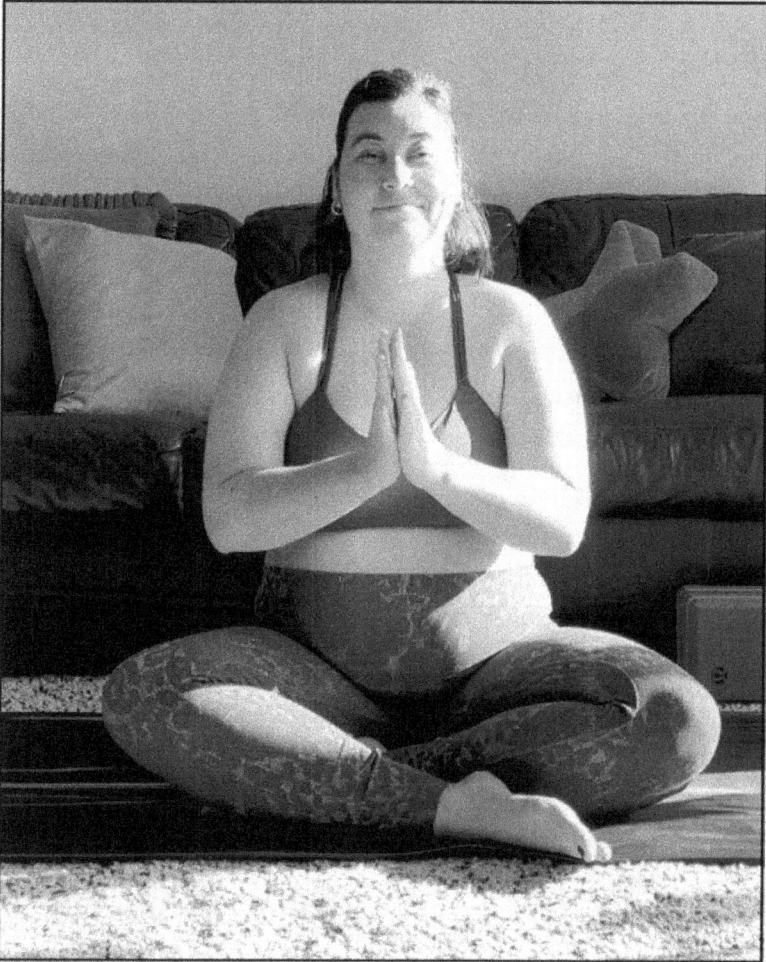

Continue for 1-2 minutes, allowing the body to settle naturally.

8.2 SELF-REGULATION TECHNIQUES FOR EMOTIONAL BALANCE

Self-regulation is like being the captain of your ship, steering through the waves of emotions that life throws at you. It's about maintaining balance and calm, even when things get stormy. Emotional self-regulation is managing your feelings so they don't control your actions or thoughts. This skill is crucial for overall well-being. When you can regulate your emotions, you respond rather than react. You make choices that align with your values, not just your impulses. This helps you navigate relationships and challenges with greater ease and grace. It enables you to stay grounded and make decisions that truly reflect your authentic self.

One powerful technique for self-regulation is biofeedback. This method helps you understand how your body responds to stress and teaches you to control those responses. Biofeedback measures heart rate, muscle tension, and skin temperature using sensors. You get real-time feedback on your physiological state. With practice, you learn to alter these signals. You may want to slow your breathing or relax your muscles. Over time, this practice helps train your body to remain calm in stressful situations. You can change your body's responses as you become more aware of them. This awareness and control enhance your ability to manage emotions effectively.

Emotional Freedom Techniques (EFT), also known as tapping, is another approach to self-regulation. It combines elements of acupuncture and psychology. You can reduce stress and negative emotions by tapping on specific points in your body. Tapping sends signals to your brain, helping it calm down. This can lower stress levels and bring about a sense of peace. EFT is simple and can be done anywhere, making it a practical tool for everyday use. It's like having a reset button for your emotions. Tapping can help you return to a state of balance and clarity when you feel overwhelmed.

Mastering self-regulation brings many benefits. When you can manage your emotions effectively, your relationships tend to improve. You communicate more clearly and listen more deeply. This fosters understanding and connection. Emotional stability also builds resilience. It helps you handle life's ups and downs with greater ease. Challenges make you more adaptable and less likely to be thrown off course. This stability creates a solid foundation for personal growth. As you navigate your emotions, you discover new strengths and insights. This journey of self-discovery can lead to a deeper understanding of yourself and your place in the world.

To practice self-regulation in daily life, start with mindful pauses. When you feel a strong emotion, pause and acknowledge it. Take a deep breath and notice what's happening in your body and mind. This creates space between feeling and reacting. It allows you to choose your response deliberately. Another helpful practice is journaling. Set aside time to write about your emotions. Reflect on what you're feeling and why. This process can reveal patterns and triggers. It helps you understand your emotional landscape better. Over time, you'll gain clarity and insight into how to manage your emotions more effectively.

Incorporating self-regulation techniques into your routine doesn't have to be complicated. Start small, and be patient with yourself. Change takes time, but each step forward builds on the last. As you practice, you'll notice shifts in how you feel and respond to situations. You'll find more calm in the chaos and more balance in change. These techniques are tools to support you on your path to emotional health. They offer a way to connect with yourself and find peace amid the noise of life.

8.3 SOMATIC EXPERIENCING TO ADDRESS TRAUMA

Picture a forest after a storm. The trees sway, and the ground shakes, but nature finds its balance again. This resilience mirrors the essence of Somatic Experiencing. This method helps heal trauma by focusing on the body's natural ability to recover and find balance. Developed by Peter Levine, this approach doesn't dive into the story of the trauma itself. Instead, it focuses on how your body reacts to stress and fear. Trauma can linger deep within your body, causing chronic stress and discomfort. Somatic experiencing taps into your body's innate wisdom, guiding you toward healing by addressing the physical responses tied to trauma.

At its core, somatic experiencing relies on several key principles. One of the most crucial is the idea of "pendulation." This involves gently moving between states of stress and calm, allowing the nervous system to find balance. By acknowledging the physical sensations that arise during stress, you can learn to release them gradually. Another important concept is "titration," where you work with small amounts of distress to avoid overwhelm. This approach allows you to process trauma slowly and safely, reducing the risk of becoming overwhelmed by intense emotions. These principles help your body regain its natural rhythm and build resilience.

To practice somatic experiencing, it's beneficial to work with a trained practitioner. They can guide you through the process, ensuring you remain safe and grounded. However, some initial exercises can be done independently. Begin by finding a quiet space where you feel at ease. Begin by noticing your breath and any sensations in your body. Pay attention to areas of tension or discomfort. Allow yourself to explore these sensations without judgment. Gradually, focus on a part of your body that feels calm or neutral. This practice encourages your body to find a balance between tension and relaxation. Repeat this process, moving between areas of discomfort and calm, allowing your body to release stored tension.

The benefits of somatic experiencing for trauma recovery are profound. Many people find that it leads to significant reductions in trauma-related symptoms. For instance, one person who experienced panic attacks found relief through these techniques. By focusing on their body's responses, they learned to manage anxiety and regain control. Another person who suffered from chronic pain discovered that addressing the physical aspects of their trauma brought about healing and comfort. These stories highlight the potential of somatic experiences to transform lives, offering a pathway to improved well-being and emotional clarity. It's a gentle yet powerful method that empowers you to reconnect with your body and emotions.

Integrating somatic experience into your healing process can enhance its effectiveness. Consider combining it with talk therapy for a comprehensive approach to trauma recovery. While somatic experiencing addresses the body's responses, talk therapy can help you process the emotional and cognitive aspects of your experience. Together, these approaches provide a holistic framework for healing. Creating a supportive environment is equally important. Surround yourself with people who understand and respect your healing journey. This support can come from friends, family, or support groups. It fosters a sense of safety and belonging, allowing you to explore your emotions and experiences without fear of judgment. In this environment, you can engage with somatic experiences and other practices in a supportive and nurturing way.

8.4 UTILIZING VISUALIZATION FOR HEALING AND GROWTH

Picture yourself in a tranquil place. Perhaps it's a forest with sunlight peeking through the leaves or a quiet beach with waves gently lapping the shore. This is where visualization begins. It's the practice of using your imagination to foster healing and growth. Visualization taps into the cognitive processes that connect your mind and body. When you visualize, your brain doesn't just see images; it also creates a mental representation of them. It also simulates the experiences associated with them. This mental imagery can influence both physical and emotional states. By imagining a peaceful scene, your brain releases calming chemicals, reducing stress and promoting relaxation. This process helps you access a deeper state of calm and clarity, making visualization a powerful tool for healing.

Advanced visualization exercises can further enhance this practice. Guided imagery is one such exercise. It involves a series of mental images designed to reduce stress and induce relaxation. You might picture yourself in a calming environment, focusing on the details around you. Imagine the gentle breeze, the sound of birds, or the sun's warmth on your skin. As you immerse yourself in this scene, your body and mind relax, easing tension and stress. Another exercise involves visualizing desired outcomes for personal growth and development. Think about a goal you want to achieve. Picture yourself accomplishing it in vivid detail. Imagine the steps you take and the feelings you experience as you reach your goal. This visualization can boost motivation and focus, guiding you toward success.

Visualization can also target specific physical ailments. Healing visualizations focus on imagining your body healing itself. If you have a sore knee, visualize warmth and light surrounding it, soothing the pain. Picture the healing process unfolding, with each breath easing the discomfort. This technique can complement other healing practices, supporting your body's healing ability.

Regular visualization practice offers long-term benefits. It can enhance focus and mental clarity, allowing you to approach tasks with a clear mind. Visualization also boosts motivation. By regularly imagining your goals, you reinforce your commitment to achieving them. This practice can even improve your ability to manage stress. As you become more adept at visualizing calming scenes, you can use this skill to center yourself in stressful situations. Over time, visualization becomes a valuable tool in your wellness routine, supporting physical and emotional health.

To create effective visualization practices, set clear intentions for each session. Know what you want to achieve: relaxation, healing, or personal growth. This intention guides your focus and enhances the effectiveness of your practice. It's also helpful to integrate visualization with meditation or breathwork. Begin with a few minutes of deep breathing to calm your mind. Then, transition into visualization, using your breath to anchor your focus. This combination deepens your experience, helping you stay engaged and present.

Chapter 8 explored advanced techniques that deepen emotional and physical healing. Like the other practices discussed, visualization offers a pathway to connect with your inner self. With practice, you can unlock new levels of awareness and healing. Next, we will explore how to tailor these exercises to meet specific needs, ensuring your practice continues to evolve and supports your well-being.

CHAPTER 9

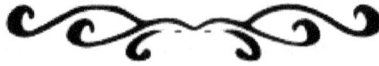

TAILORING SOMATIC EXERCISES FOR SPECIFIC NEEDS

I magine waking up each day with a nagging pain that lingers like an unwelcome shadow. Chronic pain is a silent companion for many, affecting about 20% of people worldwide (Source 1). It can make even the simplest tasks feel like climbing a mountain. Whether it's the constant ache of arthritis or the unpredictable flare-ups of fibromyalgia, chronic pain disrupts life. It seeps into your daily routine, making once enjoyable activities feel daunting. The psychological toll can be just as challenging. Living with chronic pain often leads to feelings of frustration and helplessness. It can affect your mood and make you feel isolated from others who may not understand your struggle. This emotional burden can make the pain feel even heavier.

For those living with chronic pain, finding effective management strategies is crucial. Traditional methods often focus on medication or physical therapy. While these can be helpful, somatic exercises offer a complementary approach. These exercises focus on gentle movements that increase awareness of your body's sensations. They can help reduce pain and improve mobility. Gentle stretching routines can provide relief to stiff joints. Imagine slowly extending your arms overhead and feeling the tension ease from your shoulders. These movements don't push your body to its limits. Instead, they encourage relaxation and gradual improvement. By practicing slow, controlled movements, you can minimize pain flare-ups and build confidence in your body's abilities. This approach helps you move with ease and comfort.

Consistency is key in managing chronic pain. Regular somatic practice can lead to long-term benefits. Creating a daily schedule for these exercises is essential. Start by setting aside a specific time each day. You could dedicate ten minutes to focusing on your morning routine. Use this time to reconnect with your body and address any tension. As you practice, track your pain levels and progress. You might keep a simple journal. Write down how you feel before and after each session. Over time, you'll notice patterns and improvements. These insights can guide your practice and help you make adjustments as needed.

Consider Jane's experience. For years, she lived with chronic back pain and relied heavily on medication to get through each day. After incorporating somatic exercises into her routine, she noticed a change. Her pain began to lessen, and she felt more in control. With time, she reduced her dependency on medication. This transformation gave her a sense of empowerment. She now enjoys activities she once avoided, like gardening. Her story exemplifies how somatic practices can improve daily function and well-being.

Another powerful story is that of Tom, who struggled with fibromyalgia. The unpredictability of his condition left him feeling trapped. He started a simple routine of gentle stretching each morning. Slowly, he began to notice improvements in his flexibility and energy levels. His daily functions improved, and he felt more in tune with his body. These changes brought about a renewed sense of hope. Tom's experience highlights the potential of somatic exercises to transform the lives of those with chronic pain.

Knee to Chest Hug

Lie on a mat or bed in a supported position, knees bent or legs flat out.

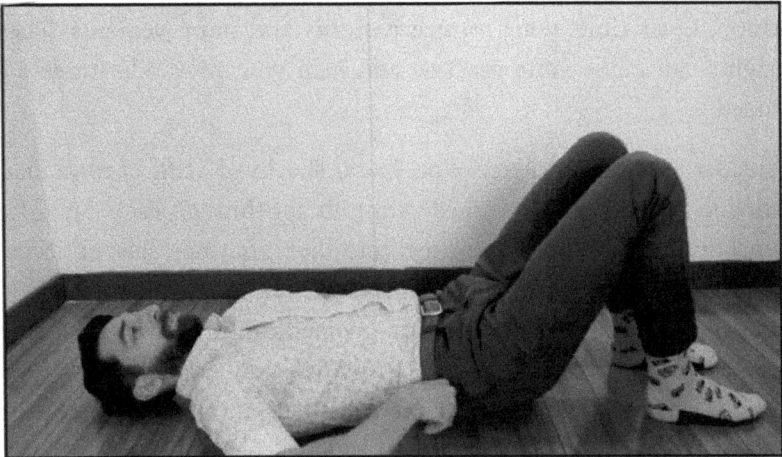

Gently hug one knee to your chest, holding behind the thigh.

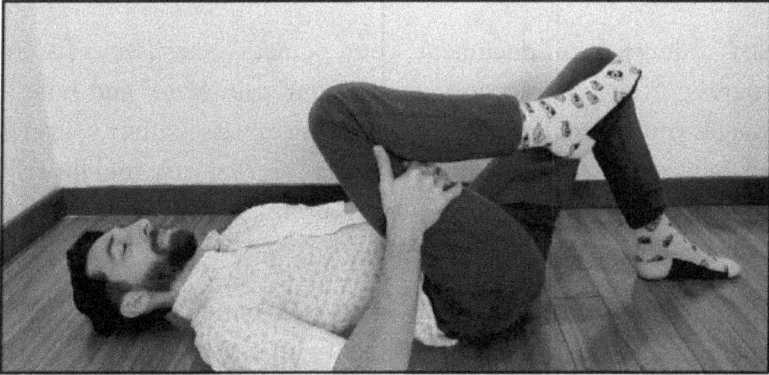

Breathe 2-3 slow breaths, then release.

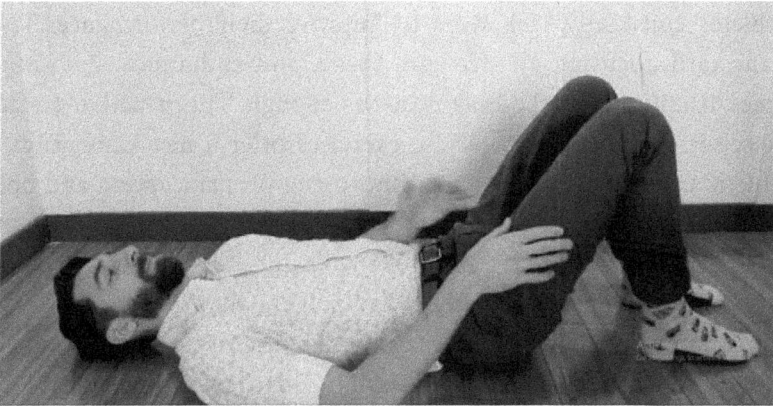

Repeat with the other leg.

Interactive Element: My Pain Management Journal

Start a journal to document your somatic exercises and track progress. After each session, record your pain levels and note any changes you experience. Record how these exercises affect your mood and daily activities. This journal can serve as a valuable tool for reflection and motivation. It will help you see your growth and remind you of the benefits of consistency.

Incorporating somatic exercises into your routine can help alleviate chronic pain. These gentle movements offer a path to healing that respects your body's limits. They promote awareness and empower you to take control of your well-being. You can transform your relationship with pain through regular practice and thoughtful reflection.

9.1 EXERCISES FOR ENHANCING ATHLETIC PERFORMANCE

Athletes constantly seek ways to improve their performance. They train hard, focusing on strength, speed, and endurance. But sometimes, traditional methods alone aren't enough. This is where somatic exercises come into play. These exercises offer a new dimension to athletic training. They focus on improving proprioception and body awareness, which are critical for any athlete. Proprioception is your body's ability to sense its position in space. It's like an internal GPS that helps you move efficiently. When you enhance this sense, you can better control your movements and reduce the risk of injury. Somatic exercises also help increase flexibility. This flexibility is crucial for preventing injuries. It allows your body to move through a full range of motion without strain. By integrating these practices, athletes can achieve better performance and resilience.

Incorporating specific somatic exercises can target various athletic goals. For athletes seeking explosive power, plyometric exercises are key. These exercises involve quick, powerful movements, such as jumps. They help build muscle strength and speed, which is essential for sports like basketball or soccer. Balance drills are another critical component. They focus on agility and coordination, which are necessary for sports that require quick direction changes. Simple exercises, such as standing on one leg or using a balance board, can help improve stability and reaction time. Core strengthening is also crucial for athletes. A strong core provides a stable base for all movements. Exercises such as planks and rotational twists can help strengthen the core. This stability supports better performance in sports ranging from running to swimming.

The benefits of incorporating somatic exercises into athletic training are numerous. Athletes often experience faster recovery times. This is because these exercises promote blood flow and reduce muscle tension. With less stress, muscles can repair more quickly. The risk of injury is also lower. As athletes become more aware of their bodies, they can avoid movements that may lead to injury. Another advantage is enhanced mental focus. Athletes who practice somatic exercises often report improved concentration during competition. This focus can make the difference between winning and losing. The exercises help clear the mind, allowing athletes to perform at their best.

Many athletes have already experienced success by incorporating somatic practices into their routines. Take Sarah, a professional runner. Adding balance drills to her training improved her agility on the track. Her enhanced coordination helped shave seconds off her race times. Similarly, a soccer player named Tom used core strengthening exercises to improve his stability during matches. The increased strength in his core enabled him to maintain balance while dribbling and tackling opponents, resulting in improved performance on the field. These stories illustrate how somatic exercises can enhance athletic performance, providing athletes with a competitive edge.

Athletes often push their bodies to the limit. They strive for excellence, seeking every possible advantage. Somatic exercises provide a unique approach to augment traditional training methods. By improving body awareness and flexibility, athletes can optimize their performance. These practices offer tangible benefits, whether through plyometric exercises for power, balance drills for agility, or core strengthening for stability. Athletes who incorporate somatic exercises into their training regimen experience improved physical well-being and enhanced mental clarity and focus. As more athletes incorporate these techniques, they reach new heights in their sports, achieving goals they once thought were unattainable.

Sit or lie down.

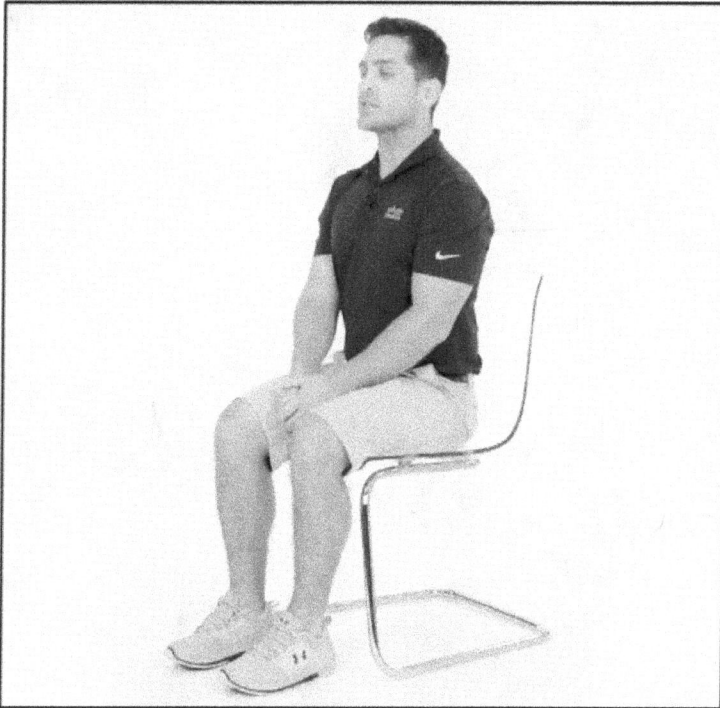

Slowly circle one ankle 3–5 times each way.

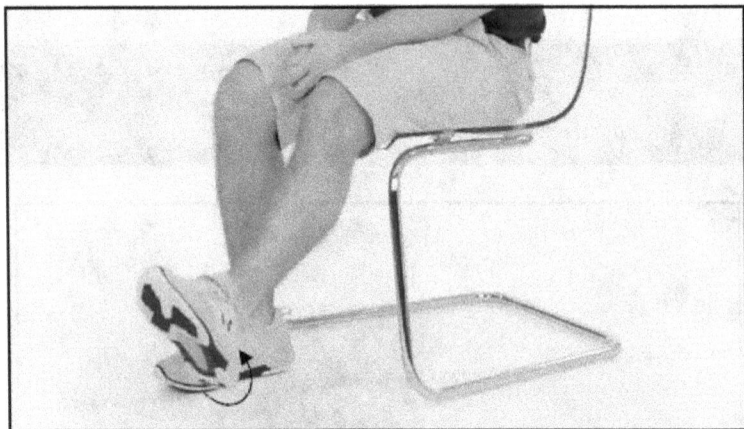

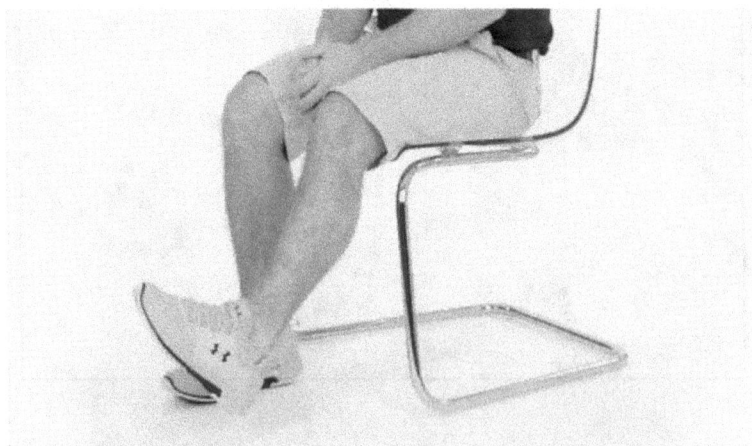

Repeat on the other side.

9.2 SOMATIC APPROACHES FOR AGE-SPECIFIC CONCERNS

As you move through different stages of life, your body has unique needs. These changes require exercises that adapt to your age. For young children, play is key. It helps them develop coordination and confidence in movement. Simple activities like playing tag or balancing games teach them to control their bodies. This builds a foundation for healthy movement patterns. Middle-aged adults often face stress and lifestyle changes. Low-impact aerobic exercises can help maintain cardiovascular health and reduce tension. They provide a way to keep active without straining the joints. For seniors, maintaining mobility and balance becomes crucial. Gentle yoga can enhance these abilities. It offers a way to stretch and strengthen muscles without injury. These activities not only improve physical health but also boost mental well-being.

Flexibility and strength are essential at any age. As you get older, muscles and joints lose some of their elasticity. This can lead to stiffness and discomfort. Regular somatic exercises can counteract these effects. They encourage your body to move more fluidly. This reduces the risk of falls and injuries. Exercises like gentle stretching routines help maintain the range of motion. They keep muscles flexible and joints lubricated. Strength exercises, even at a low intensity, help maintain muscle mass. This is particularly important for daily activities such as climbing stairs or carrying groceries. A consistent routine can lead to increased independence. It allows older adults to enjoy life without depending on others for basic tasks.

The benefits of somatic practice extend beyond physical health. They include enhanced cognitive functions, such as memory and attention. When you engage in activities that require coordination and concentration, your brain forms new connections. This helps keep your mind sharp. For instance, seniors who practice gentle yoga may find that they remember things more effectively. A middle-aged adult participating in low-impact aerobics may notice an improvement in focus at work. These exercises stimulate the brain, promoting mental agility and acuity. It's a simple way to support your body and mind as you age. Regular practice also fosters a sense of accomplishment. It builds confidence in your ability to stay active and maintain good health.

Consider the story of Helen, a senior who began practicing yoga in her 70s. She was hesitant at first, worried about her balance. But over time, she found that her confidence grew. She could move with more ease and less fear of falling. Her story is not unique. Many seniors have found that somatic exercises allow them to maintain active lifestyles. They enjoy hobbies like gardening or walking with friends. Parents often notice changes when they engage children in somatic play. Kids become more coordinated and less prone to accidents. They also gain a better understanding of their bodies.

Lifelong somatic practice can transform your experience of aging. It keeps you connected to your body and aware of its needs. This awareness enables you to adapt to changes and maintain your overall well-being. Whether through playful activities for kids, aerobic exercises for adults, or yoga for seniors, somatic techniques offer something for everyone. They provide a way to stay active and engaged at any age. These practices help you enjoy life more fully, regardless of the challenges that aging might bring.

Somatic Core Twist

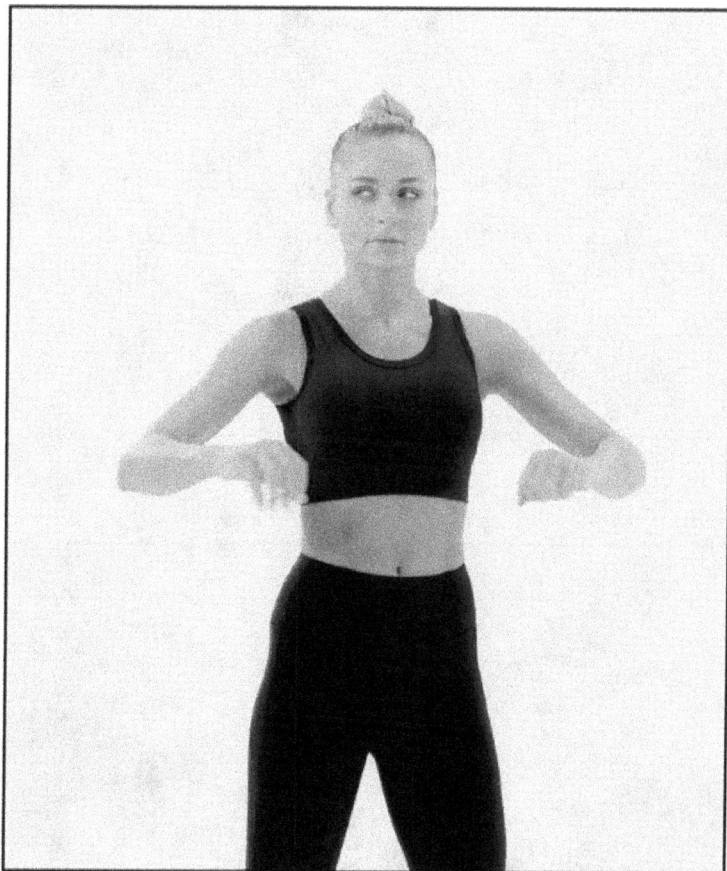

Stand tall with feet hip-width apart and knees slightly bent.

○—• Slowly twist your torso side to side, keeping your hips stable.

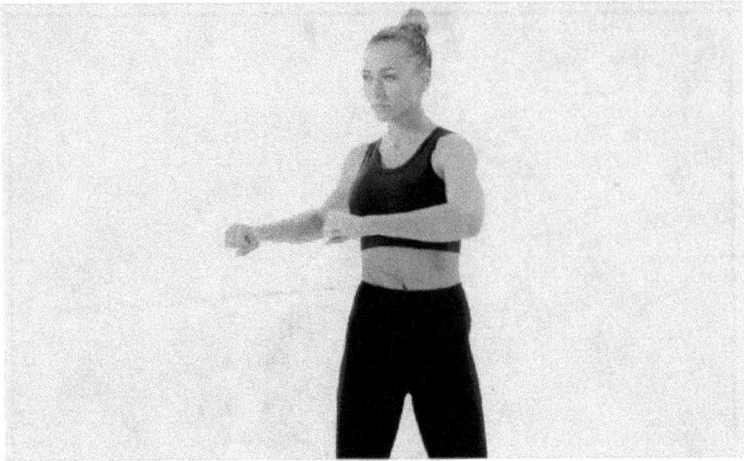

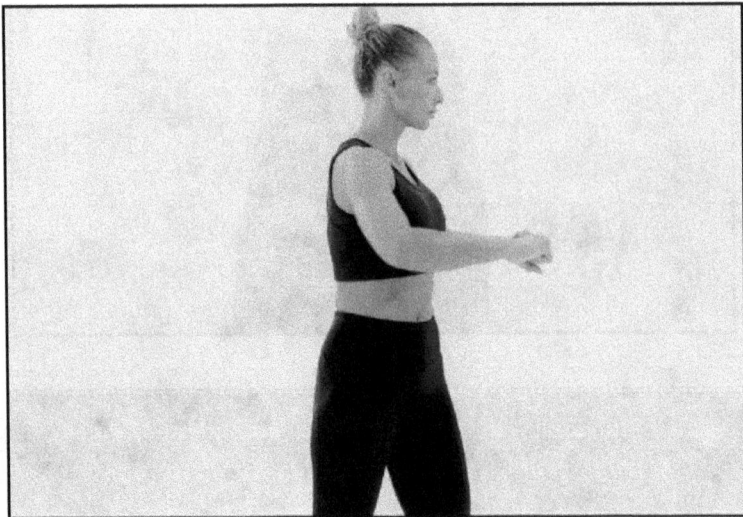

9.3 CREATING A PERSONALIZED SOMATIC EXERCISE PLAN

Personalization in somatic practice is the key to unlocking its true potential. By tailoring a routine to fit your unique goals and abilities, you make the exercises work for you. Everyone's body is different, and what works for one person might not suit another. This is why personal preferences play a huge role in your success. When you enjoy and relate to what you're doing, you're more likely to stick with it. Adherence becomes more manageable, and the likelihood of achieving tangible results increases. Your goals might be to reduce stress, improve flexibility, or feel more connected to your body. Whatever they are, identifying them clearly will help guide your practice. Consider your goal and how somatic exercises can help support it.

To create a personalized somatic plan, assess your current physical condition. Be honest about any limitations or areas that need extra attention. This might include past injuries or specific areas of weakness. Once you have a clear picture, you can select exercises that align with your objectives. If improving flexibility is your goal, focus on stretches that target tight muscles. For stress relief, incorporate breathing exercises that promote relaxation and calmness. Tailoring your routine to your needs ensures that each session is meaningful and effective. Next, set realistic practice goals. Determine how often you want to practice and for how long. Start small, with ten minutes daily, and gradually increase as you become more comfortable.

The benefits of a customized somatic routine are numerous. When exercises are tailored to your needs, you experience greater satisfaction and results. This personalization leads to increased motivation and engagement. You feel more connected to the practice because it addresses your needs and goals directly. Rapid achievement of personal health goals becomes possible when the exercises align with your goals. You see progress faster, which reinforces your commitment to the practice. This positive cycle of motivation and progress creates a sense of empowerment. You realize you have the tools to improve your well-being, which fuels further dedication.

Consider the story of Emily, who wanted to improve her posture and reduce neck tension. She worked long hours at a desk, and this goal was essential to her daily comfort. She personalized her routine by incorporating specific neck stretches and core strengthening exercises. Within a few weeks, she noticed a significant improvement in her posture and a reduction in tension in her neck. Her success didn't end there. Inspired by her progress, she added more exercises to her routine, targeting other areas of her body. This personalized approach enabled her to transform her lifestyle, achieving goals she once thought were unattainable.

John's journey exemplifies the transformative power of personalized somatic exercises for those juggling demanding schedules. As a devoted father and career-oriented individual, John faced the common challenge of integrating regular physical activity into his already packed day. Recognizing the importance of maintaining his health for his family and professional life, he created a somatic exercise plan that could seamlessly blend into his routine without overwhelming it. Starting with a clear assessment of his available time and specific health objectives, John pinpointed that his primary goals were to enhance his overall energy levels and improve his focus—critical components for his demanding job and active family life. He meticulously selected exercises that were efficient and could be performed in short bursts, and required minimal equipment, ensuring that he could easily undertake them at home or even in his office. John's routine consisted of dynamic stretches to awaken his body in the morning and mindful breathing techniques designed to center his focus before diving into his day. These practices took no more than ten minutes, yet the impact was profound. He also incorporated brief midday sessions, which involved chair-based somatic movements to relieve the tension built up from hours of sitting. In the evenings, John dedicated a slightly more extended period to engaging in comprehensive exercises that focused on core strength, flexibility, and relaxation, preparing his body and mind for restful sleep. This strategic approach enabled John to remain committed to his practice, overcoming the time constraint without compromising the quality of his exercise routine. Remarkably, the benefits extended beyond physical well-being. John discovered that these mindful, somatic sessions significantly boosted his mental clarity and concentration, enabling him to tackle his professional responsibilities with enhanced vigor and creativity. Moreover, the increased energy levels and stress management positively influenced his interactions with his family, fostering a more joyful and connected home environment. John's story vividly illustrates that with thoughtful planning and a commitment to personal well-being, the obstacles of time and a busy lifestyle can be surmounted. By tailoring the somatic exercises to fit his specific circumstances and needs, John achieved his health goals and experienced profound improvements in his daily life, demonstrating the life-changing potential of a personalized somatic practice. Creating a personalized somatic exercise plan is not just about choosing the correct movements. It's about crafting a practice that resonates with you. It encourages you to listen to your body and respond to its needs. Through this approach, you find a deeper connection to your well-being. You develop a routine that fits seamlessly into your life, making it a sustainable part of your daily routine. The flexibility and adaptability of somatic exercises make them a valuable tool for anyone seeking to enhance their overall well-being. Focusing on what matters most to you creates a pathway to greater satisfaction and success.

Balance Drill

Add a balance challenge — lift one heel or one foot slightly as you twist. Hold both ends of a cloth to help with balance.

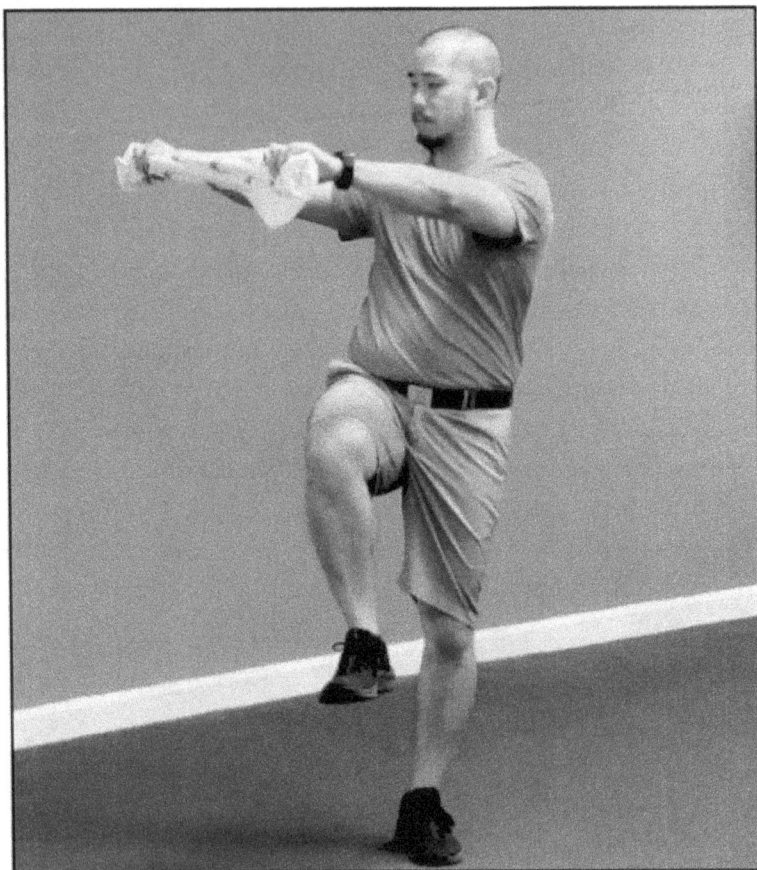

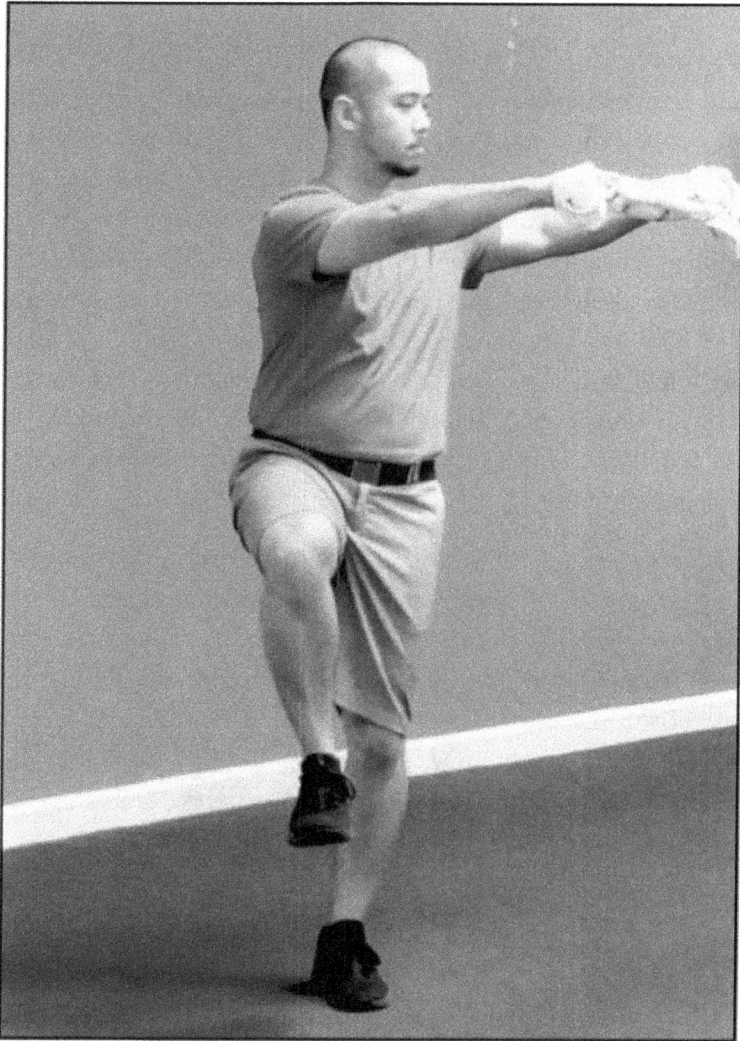

Repeat for 8-10 slow, controlled rounds,   breathing
steadily throughout.

Certain groups benefit significantly from exercises tailored to their unique needs in the diverse wellness landscape. Individuals with disabilities, for instance, often face barriers that can limit their access to typical exercise routines. Wheelchair users, for example, may find traditional exercises challenging. Yet, somatic practices offer a way to engage and strengthen their bodies without the need for standing or balance. By focusing on seated exercises, they can improve their strength and flexibility. Gentle arm stretches and torso twists can be performed while seated, helping to enhance circulation and mobility. These adaptations ensure that everyone can participate, regardless of physical limitations.

Pregnant women and new mothers also have distinct exercise needs. During pregnancy, the body undergoes significant changes, making some movements uncomfortable or unsafe. Prenatal yoga becomes a valuable tool, offering modifications that accommodate a growing belly and shifting center of gravity. These exercises focus on gentle stretching and strengthening, supporting the back and hips. Deep breathing techniques can also help manage stress and prepare for childbirth. After childbirth, new mothers can utilize modified exercises to regain strength and balance. Simple core exercises, done slowly and carefully, can help restore muscle tone after childbirth, supporting recovery and well-being.

Exercise might seem daunting for people with chronic illnesses or limited mobility. Low-impact exercises become essential, as they minimize stress on the body while promoting health. Individuals with cardiovascular concerns, for instance, can benefit from exercises that raise the heart rate gently without undue strain. Walking, swimming, or even chair-based movements can improve cardiovascular health while being safe. These exercises help maintain fitness levels and improve quality of life. They provide a way to stay active and engaged with the body, even when facing health challenges.

Inclusive somatic practices foster a supportive environment for all. By adapting exercises, we increase accessibility and participation. This inclusivity empowers individuals, providing them with the tools to engage meaningfully with their bodies. It fosters a sense of independence, enabling individuals to take charge of their health and well-being. When exercises are tailored to individual needs, practitioners feel seen and valued. This recognition encourages continued practice and engagement, leading to improved health outcomes.

The stories of those who have benefited from adapted somatic exercises are inspiring. Consider Linda, who uses a wheelchair. She found that seated exercises helped her improve her upper body strength and flexibility. This improvement has enhanced her daily function and increased her independence. Linda reports feeling more energetic and capable, enjoying activities she once found exhausting. Similarly, Sarah, a mother of two, maintained her fitness during pregnancy with prenatal yoga. She found that the adapted exercises eased her back pain and prepared her for childbirth. Postpartum, she continued with gentle core exercises to help her regain strength and confidence. Her story highlights the power of somatic exercises to support mothers during a significant life transition.

Adapting somatic exercises for special populations reflects a commitment to inclusivity and empowerment. It recognizes that, regardless of physical ability or life stage, everyone deserves access to practices that support health and well-being. These exercises open doors to improved quality of life by providing tailored options. They offer a pathway to greater confidence, independence, and joy in movement. These practices remind us that wellness is for everyone, and with the proper adaptations, we can all find ways to engage with our bodies and enhance our lives.

CHAPTER 10

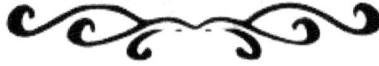

SUSTAINING LONG-TERM TRANSFORMATION AND GROWTH

I magine standing in front of a mirror, not just to check your appearance, but to see yourself as you truly are. You observe not just your reflection but the journey you've taken, the progress you've made, and the areas that still need attention. This moment of reflection is more than just a glance; it is a deep dive into your experiences, a chance to understand your growth, and a way to chart your future path. Reflection, in this sense, becomes a powerful tool in your somatic practice. It allows you to pause, evaluate, and learn from your experiences. This is crucial for sustaining long-term transformation and growth.

Reflection is not just about thinking back on what you've done; it's also about learning from your experiences. It's about understanding how those experiences have shaped you and what they can teach you moving forward. By regularly reflecting on your somatic exercises, you can deepen your understanding of the exercises themselves and how your body and mind respond to them. This understanding can sustain your interest and commitment over time. When you reflect, you begin to see patterns in your practice. You may notice that specific exercises make you feel more relaxed, while others energize you. Recognizing these patterns can help you identify what works best for you and pinpoint areas that require more focus.

Growth is not always linear, and reflection can help you see the non-linear paths that have contributed to your development. By looking back at where you started and noting your progress, you can appreciate how far you've come. This appreciation fuels your motivation to continue. Reflection can also reveal areas where you might be stuck or where you could improve. You may have hit a plateau or haven't tried new exercises. Reflecting on these aspects can highlight areas for further development and inspire you to explore new techniques or revisit old ones with fresh eyes.

To incorporate reflection into your regular practice, consider using several methods. One effective technique is to keep a reflective journal. This journal becomes a personal space where you document your experiences, noting what you did, how it felt, and what you learned. You can also use it to explore physical and emotional changes, writing about how specific exercises affect your mood or body. Over time, this journal becomes a rich resource, offering insights into your growth and helping you set new goals.

Guided prompts can enhance your reflective practice by encouraging deeper exploration. For example, prompts might ask you to describe a recent exercise session in detail, focusing on the sensations and emotions you experienced during that session. They also prompt you to consider how your practice aligns with your personal goals. By responding to these prompts, you engage more fully with your practice, uncovering insights that might otherwise remain hidden.

Reflective practice offers several benefits that can enhance self-awareness and promote continuous improvement. By reflecting, you gain increased clarity on your personal goals. You understand what you want to achieve and why it matters to you. This clarity allows you to align your practice with your broader life objectives, making each session more meaningful. You also develop a greater appreciation of your progress over time. This appreciation helps you stay motivated, especially when challenges arise. You see that every small step counts, contributing to your overall transformation.

Let's consider some practical examples of implementing reflection in your practice. Set aside time each month for a reflection session. During this time, revisit your journal and note any patterns or changes that you observe. Ask yourself questions like, "What have I learned this month?" or "What areas need more attention?" This monthly review helps you stay on track and adjust your practice as needed. Another method is to create a visual progress map. This map could take the form of a chart or diagram, showing your achievements and milestones. You might mark when you mastered a new exercise or noticed a significant change in your flexibility or mood. Seeing your progress visually can be motivating and affirming, reinforcing the value of your efforts.

Mirror Awareness Exercise

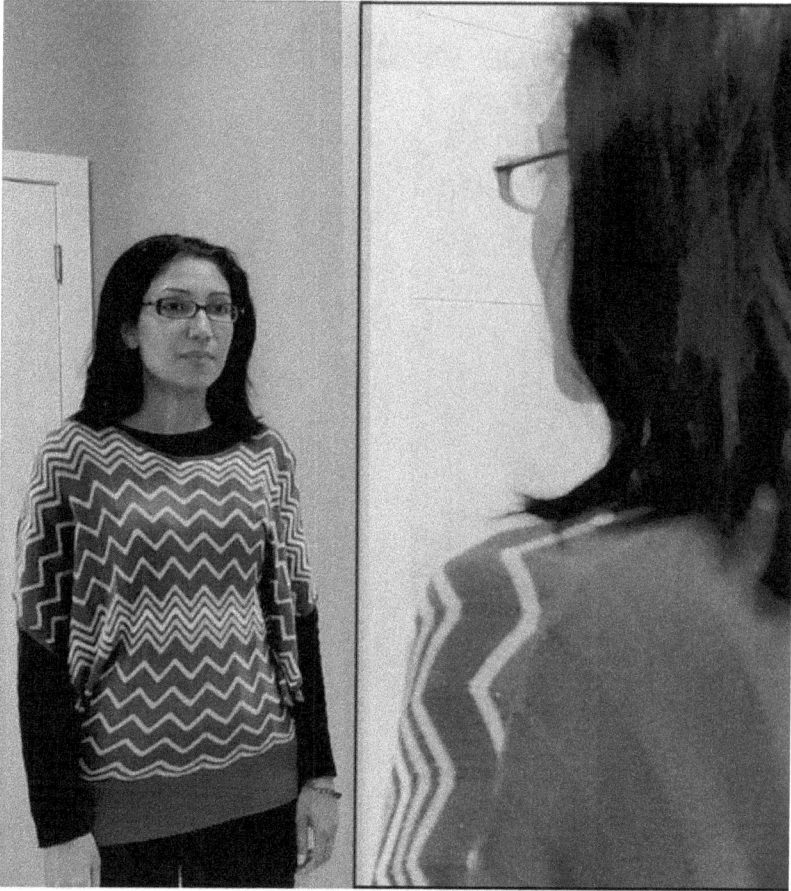

Look into a mirror and gently make eye contact with yourself.

Say one kind affirmation out loud (e.g. "I am enough.").

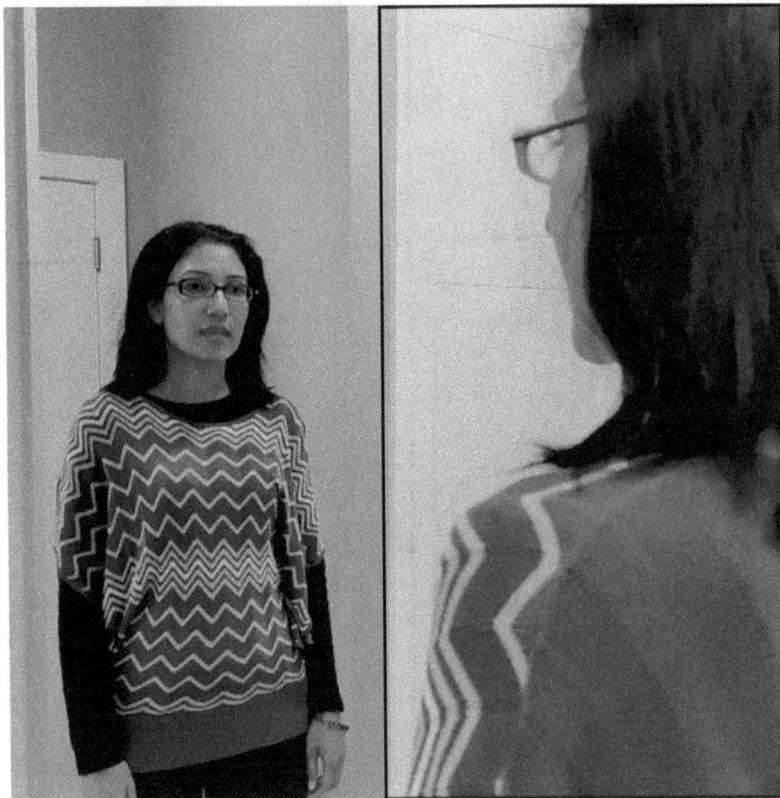

Take one   slow breath,   affirming kindness   toward
yourself.

Reflective Practices to Try:

- **Monthly Reflection Sessions**: Schedule a time to review your journal and assess your progress. Use this time to realign your goals and celebrate achievements.
- **Visual Progress Map**: Create a chart or diagram to track milestones and achievements visually. Update it regularly to see your progress at a glance.

Engaging in reflective practices enhances your self-awareness and fosters a deeper understanding of your physical and mental states. This process of introspection makes you more sensitive to the nuanced changes your body and mind undergo during your exercises, granting you the clarity needed to make well-informed decisions regarding the future direction of your practice. Reflection transcends mere recollection of past actions; it serves as a proactive tool that equips you with the power to sculpt your somatic journey with insight and deliberation. Through this ongoing interplay of contemplation and action, you can sustain continuing transformation and growth, ultimately leading to a balanced and enriching practice. By systematically reviewing and assessing your progress, you'll uncover patterns and insights that guide your practice to evolve in alignment with your changing needs and goals, ensuring a dynamic and responsive approach to personal well-being. Embracing Change: Adapting Your Practice Over Time

Change is a constant in life. It can come unexpectedly or slowly unfold over time. In the context of somatic practice, change is something you must accept and work with. Your body, your mind, and your life circumstances all evolve. These shifts require adjustments in how you approach your exercises. Sticking rigidly to the same routine might seem comforting, but it can limit your growth. Instead, embracing change and adapting your practice can lead to more extraordinary transformation and healing.

Life changes can have a significant impact on your practice. You might change jobs, move to a new city, or experience changes in your health. These shifts can disrupt your routine and challenge your commitment. You might find it hard to maintain the same intensity or frequency of practice. That's okay. It's normal for your practice to ebb and flow with life's demands. The key is to stay flexible and adjust your practice to fit your current situation. You may start with shorter sessions or choose exercises that match your energy levels. By adapting in this way, you remain engaged without overwhelming yourself.

Your goals can also change over time. Initially, focus on alleviating physical pain or stress. However, as you progress, you may become interested in exploring emotional awareness or enhancing flexibility. These evolving goals can shape your somatic practice, guiding you to try new exercises or techniques. Adapting your practice to align with your goals ensures that your efforts remain meaningful and satisfying. It keeps your practice fresh and relevant to your needs.

To adapt your practice effectively, consider adjusting both the intensity and duration of your exercises. On days when you feel energetic, you may opt for a more extended session with more challenging movements. A gentle routine might be more appropriate on days when your energy is low. This flexibility allows you to honor your body's needs while engaging in meaningful practice. You may also explore new exercises that address emerging interests or challenges. To build strength, incorporate resistance exercises. If you're interested in emotional exploration, try intuitive movement or guided visualization.

A flexible approach to somatic practice offers several benefits. It helps you avoid burnout by preventing your routine from becoming monotonous. When you're open to change, you maintain enthusiasm and motivation. This openness fosters creativity and exploration in your practice. You become curious about new ways to move and feel, which can lead to unexpected discoveries. By staying adaptable, you ensure that your practice continues to nourish and support you, no matter what life throws your way.

Change can be daunting, but it also presents growth opportunities. When encountering challenges, try to view them as chances to learn and evolve. Setting new intentions with each phase of life can help you stay focused and motivated. These intentions serve as a guiding light, reminding you of what you hope to achieve through your practice. They keep you grounded and aligned with your deeper values and desires.

Viewing change as an opportunity rather than a setback can transform your perspective. Instead of resisting change, embrace it as a natural part of your practice. Each shift becomes a stepping stone toward greater awareness and understanding. Change invites you to explore new possibilities and deepen your connection with yourself. It encourages you to grow and transform, both in your practice and life.

As you adapt your practice over time, you'll likely encounter periods of uncertainty or doubt. Questioning whether you're on the right path or making progress is a natural and expected part of the process. During these moments, remind yourself that growth isn't always linear. Sometimes, it takes a few steps back to move forward. Trust in the process, and remember that every change, no matter how small, contributes to your overall transformation.

Incorporating change into your somatic practice requires patience and self-compassion. Be gentle with yourself as you navigate new terrain. Celebrate the small victories and acknowledge the lessons learned from setbacks. Each experience, whether positive or challenging, adds depth and richness to your practice. This depth enhances your understanding of yourself and your body, enabling you to navigate life with greater ease and resilience.

By embracing change and adapting your practice, you create a dynamic and evolving experience. This approach supports your physical and emotional well being, enriching your life in the process. It encourages you to remain open and curious, ready to explore whatever comes next. This way, change becomes a powerful ally in your journey toward lasting transformation and growth.

Reflection Pause (3-Minute Reset)

Gentle Somatic Yoga

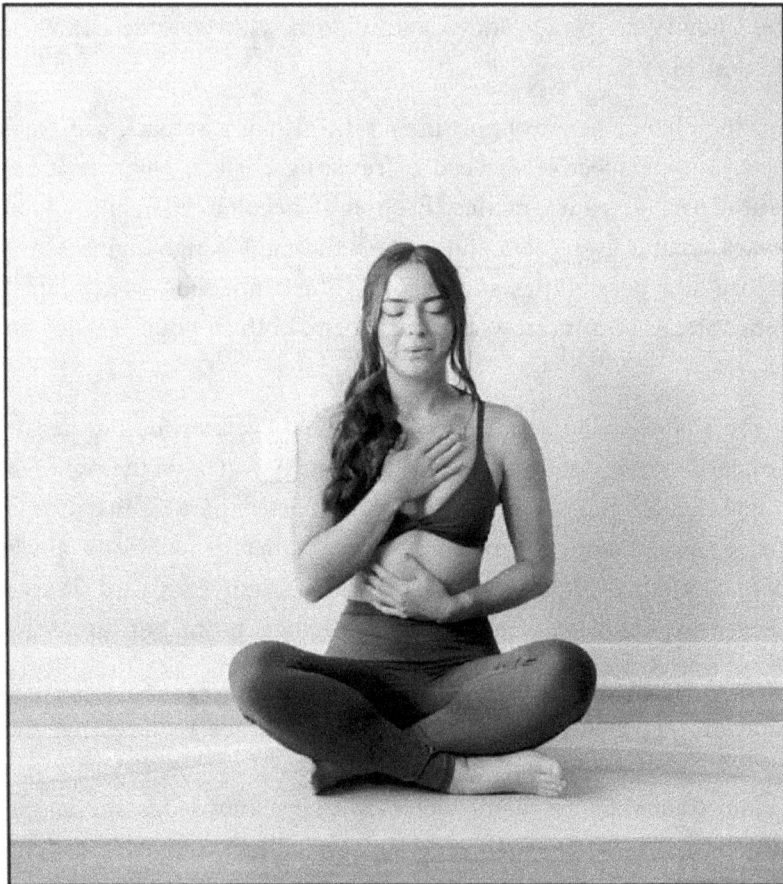

Sit quietly and take a slow breath in and out.

Breathe slowly in through the nose.

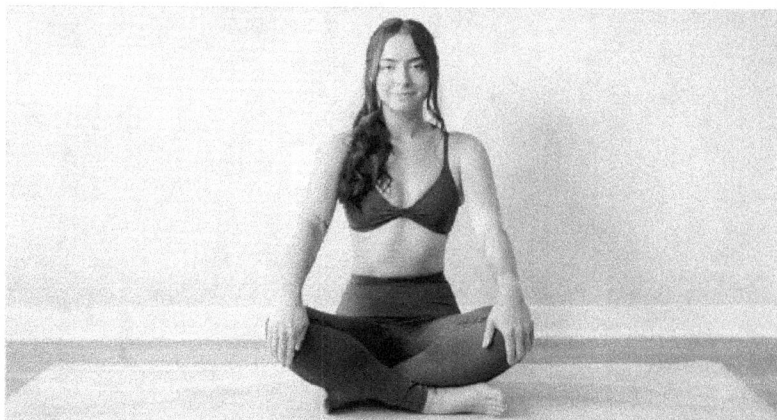

Add gentle movement — shoulder roll, neck release, or sway.

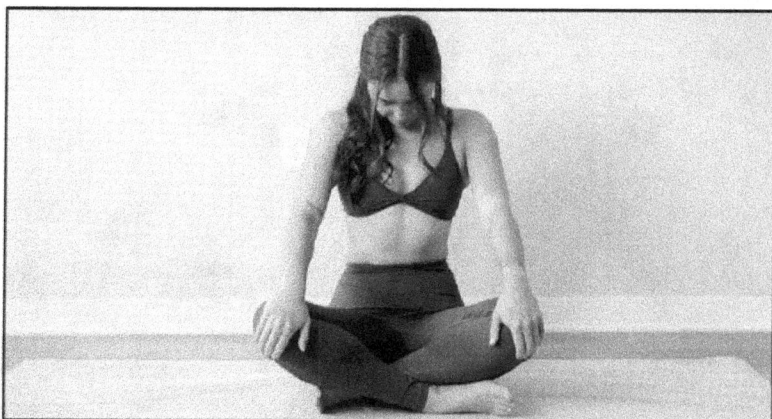

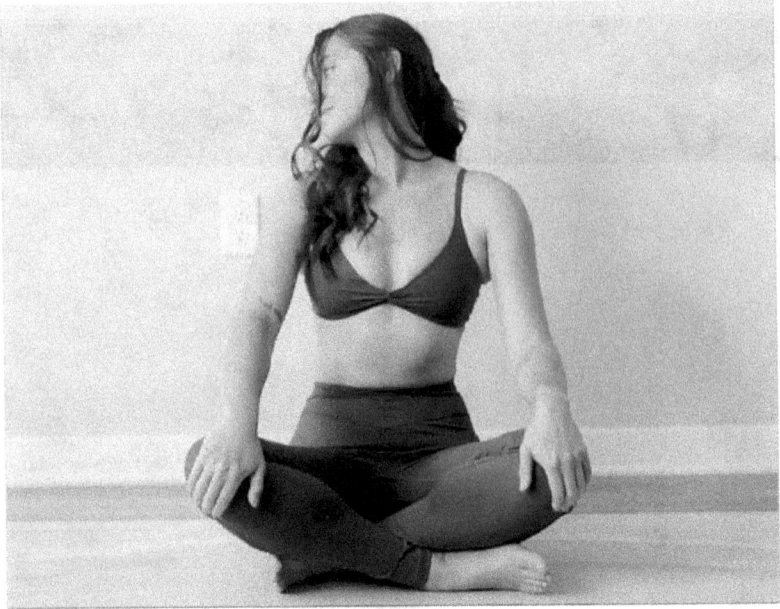

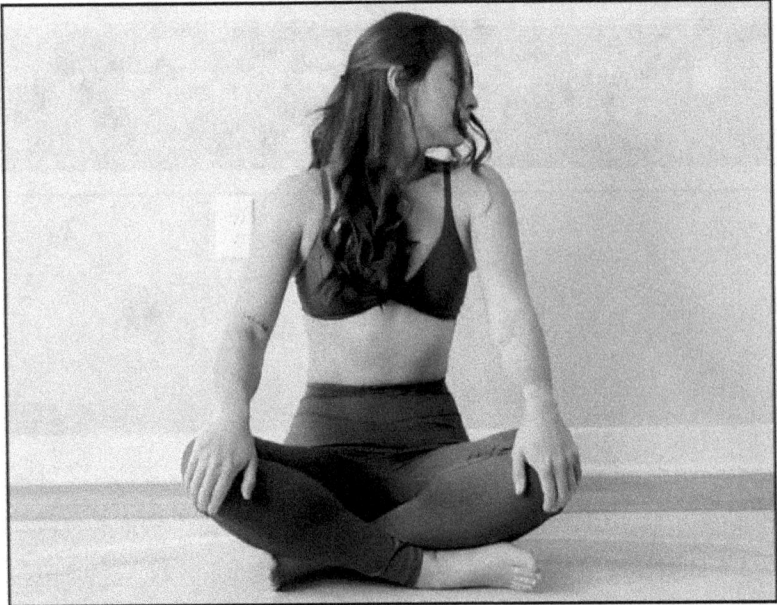

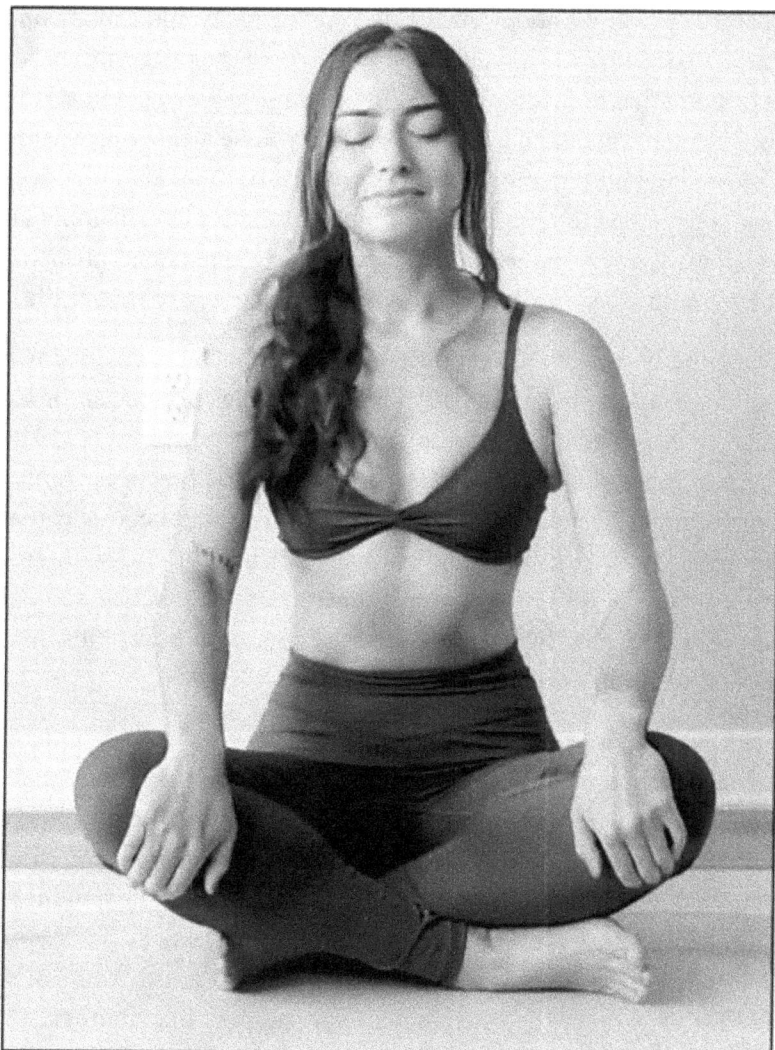

○•➤ Scan your body briefly,   then finish with one deep
breath.

10.1 CONTINUING YOUR SOMATIC JOURNEY: LIFELONG LEARNING AND GROWTH

Imagine a garden that grows as long as you tend to it, bringing new blooms and fruits each season. This is how I see lifelong learning in somatic practice. It's about nurturing your curiosity and staying open to new experiences. This openness keeps your practice vibrant and full of potential. It encourages you to continue exploring and seeking new ways to understand and connect with yourself. Lifelong learning isn't just about adding more exercises to your routine. It's about deepening your understanding of the connections between your mind and body. This deeper understanding is what drives personal growth. It allows you to see your practice as a living, evolving part of your life.

One of the best ways to continue learning in somatic practice is by attending workshops or retreats. These gatherings provide an opportunity to learn advanced techniques and gain new insights. They provide a focused time to dive deeper into specific practices. You can learn from experienced teachers and connect with others who share your interests. Workshops and retreats can inspire you with fresh ideas and perspectives. They can re-energize your practice and help you see it in a new light. You'll return home with new skills and a renewed sense of purpose.

Exploring related disciplines can also enrich your somatic practice. Practices such as tai chi or yoga offer alternative approaches to movement and awareness. They can complement your somatic exercises by providing new tools and techniques to enhance your practice. Each discipline's focus and philosophy can broaden your understanding of health and well-being. Exploring these related practices gives you a broader perspective on nurturing your body and mind. You can see how different practices interconnect and support one another. This exploration can lead to a more holistic approach to your well-being.

Continuous growth through lifelong learning leads to more profound personal transformation and fulfillment. As you learn and grow, you enhance your understanding of the mind-body connection. You become more aware of how your physical and mental processes influence each other. This awareness allows you to make more informed choices about your practice and life. You gain a greater sense of control and empowerment. Your practice becomes a source of strength and balance. It supports you in facing life's challenges with resilience and grace.

Ongoing learning also offers a broader perspective on health and well-being. You begin to see that well-being is not just about physical fitness. It's about finding harmony between your body and mind. It's also about nurturing your emotional and spiritual well-being. This broader perspective encourages you to explore new paths and possibilities. It invites you to see your practice as a journey that evolves and grows with you.

Consider the story of Alex, who began his somatic practice in search of relief from chronic back pain. He started with simple exercises, focusing on movement and awareness. Over time, he attended workshops and explored yoga, which offered new insights. These experiences deepened his understanding of his body and mind. He discovered how interconnected his physical and emotional health were. This realization led to personal breakthroughs. Alex found new ways to manage stress and improve his overall well-being. His journey illustrates the power of lifelong learning in somatic practice. It shows how continuous growth can lead to profound transformation.

Another example is Lisa, who found joy in collaborating with others through community involvement. She joined a local somatic group and began attending regular classes. Through these connections, she learned from diverse perspectives and experiences. She collaborated on projects and shared her insights. This community involvement enriched her practice and expanded her understanding. Lisa's story highlights how collaboration and community can enhance lifelong learning. It shows how sharing our journeys can lead to greater fulfillment and growth.

Remember to stay curious as you embark on a lifelong learning journey in your somatic practice. Let your curiosity guide you to new experiences and discoveries. Be open to exploring new techniques and approaches. Each new experience adds depth and richness to your practice. It helps you grow and evolve, both as a professional and as an individual. Lifelong learning is a journey without an endpoint. It's about constantly seeking growth and transformation. It's about finding new ways to connect with yourself and the world.

MAKE A DIFFERENCE
WITH YOUR REVIEW

UNLOCK THE POWER OF GENEROSITY

"Money can't buy happiness, but giving it away can."

— FREDDIE MERCURY

You've reached the final page—thank you for walking this journey with me. Each gentle movement, each breath of awareness, brings you closer to calm, balance, and ease.

Now, I'd like to ask one last favor. Would you help someone just like you—curious about *At Home Somatic Therapy Exercises for Beginners: Easy & Gentle Movements for Nervous System Regulation, Emotional Healing and Lasting Calm* but unsure where to start?

My mission is to make somatic therapy simple, practical, and healing for everyone. But to reach more people, I need your help.

Most people choose books based on reviews. Your honest words can guide another beginner toward greater peace.

It costs nothing and takes less than a minute, but your review could change someone's somatic journey. Your words could help...

- one more person ease stress at the end of a long day.
- one more beginner feel confident trying gentle movements.
- one more reader discover peace in their body and mind.
- one more person reduce tension and improve their sleep.
- one more life touched by calm and healing.

To leave a review, simply scan the QR code below or visit this link:

https://www.amazon.com/review/review-your-purchases/?asin=B0G4JFRSC2

If you love helping others, you're my kind of person.

Thank you from the bottom of my heart!

S.C. Monroe

CONCLUSION

Throughout this book, I've shared the incredible potential of somatic exercises. My goal has been to make these practices accessible and beneficial for everyone. I want you to see how they can enhance body awareness, relieve tension, and promote overall well-being.

We've explored so many key points together. We started by understanding the foundations of somatic exercises. You learned about the science behind them and how they differ from traditional workouts. We then moved on to creating beginner-friendly routines and integrating these exercises into your busy life.

As we progressed, you discovered how to address stress, anxiety, and tension through somatic practices. You learned gentle flow routines, strength recovery techniques, and exercises that focus on balance and alignment. We also discussed how to tailor these practices for specific needs, such as chronic pain management, athletic performance, and age-related concerns.

The main takeaway I want you to remember is this: somatic therapy exercises can transform your physical and emotional health. They offer a path to healing and growth you can follow throughout life. You can achieve meaningful results by committing to regular practice and applying the strategies you've learned.

It's important to reflect on your progress and personalize your practice as you go. Your needs and goals will change over time, and that's okay. Adapt your routines to suit your current stage in the journey. Keep exploring and learning about somatic therapy exercises and related disciplines. There's always more to discover.

Remember, you're not alone in this journey. Connect with others who share your interests. Join online forums or local groups. A supportive community can make a big difference in your practice and motivation.

As we come to the end of this book, I want to leave you with a call to action: Take the first steps toward integrating somatic exercises into your life. Start small, but start today. These practices offer greater mobility, less stress, and a deeper connection between your mind and body.

I believe in you. I know you have the power to achieve incredible transformation and healing through these practices. Trust in the process and yourself. Every small step you take is toward a healthier, happier you.

My journey with somatic therapy exercises has been life-changing. They've helped me overcome physical pain and emotional challenges and given me a new appreciation for my body and its wisdom. I want you to experience those same benefits.

So, keep exploring, keep practicing, and keep growing. The path to well-being is a lifelong journey, but it's one filled with incredible rewards. I'm honored to be a part of your journey, and I look forward to seeing where it takes you.

Remember, you have everything you need within you to succeed. Your body is your most excellent guide. Listen to, respect, and nourish it through the power of somatic exercises.

Thank you for joining me on this journey. I wish you all the best as you continue to explore, learn, and grow. Keep shining, my friend. The world needs your light.

With love and gratitude,

S.C. Monroe

REFERENCES

- *Neuroscience of Somatic Psychology* https://www.somatopia.com/blog/ neuroscience-somatic-techniques
- *Proprioception: The Sixth Sense & Activities To Help Regulate* https://www. communicationclubhouse.com/blog/proprioception-the-sixth-sense/#:~: text=Aside%20from%20supporting%20a% 20good,or%20learn%20a%20new%20dance.
- *Somatic experiencing – effectiveness and key factors of a ...* https://pmc.ncbi.nlm. nih.gov/articles/PMC8276649/#:~:text=Results%3A%20Findings% 20provide%20preliminary%20evidence,traumatized%20and%20non%2D- traumatized%20samples.
- *Neuroscience of Somatic Psychology* https://www.somatopia.com/blog/ neuroscience-somatic-techniques
- *Somatic Stretching: How It Works, Benefits, and Starter ...* https://www. everydayhealth.com/fitness/what-is-somatic-stretching/
- *Somatic Experiencing Therapy: 10 Best Exercises 6 ...* https://positivepsychology. com/somatic-experiencing/
- *12 Effective Somatic Therapy Exercises for Holistic Healing* https://www. monakirstein.com/somatic-therapy-exercises/
- *Coping with stress at work* https://www.apa.org/topics/healthy-workplaces/ work-stress
- *Buddhist Antecedents to the Body Scan Meditation* https://www. buddhismuskunde.uni-hamburg.de/pdf/5-personen/analayo/ buddhistantecedentsbodyscan.pdf
- *The Role of Movement in Emotional Healing* https://www.coreenergetics.org/ the-role-of-movement-in-emotional-healing/
- *Mindful Movement: How It's Done and Why It's Good for You* https://www. fitnessblender.com/articles/mindful-movement-how-it-s-done-and-why-it- s-good-for-you
- *Somatic Visualizing: How and Why It Works* https://www.edgemagazine.net/ 2008/03/somatic-visualizing-how-and-why-it-works/
- *Breathing Practices for Stress and Anxiety Reduction* https://pmc.ncbi.nlm.nih. gov/articles/PMC10741869/#:~:text=Breathing% 20practices'%20effects%20on%20the,intrin- sic%20to%20stress%20and%20anxiety.
- *Grounding the Connection Between Psyche and Soma* https://pmc.ncbi.nlm.nih. gov/articles/PMC7982724/
- *10 Easy Somatic Exercises for Stress & Tension Relief* https://uncovercounseling. com/blog/10-easy-somatic-exercises-to-relieve-stress-and-tension/

- *Consistent Bedtime Routines are Linked to Better Sleep ...* https://aquila.usm.edu/cgi/viewcontent.cgi?article=29646context=dissertations
- *Dynamic vs. Static Stretching: Is One Better?* https://health.clevelandclinic.org/dynamic-stretching-vs-static-stretching
- *Somatic Exercise and Trauma Recovery* https://acrm.org/rehabilitation-medicine/somatic-exercises-and-trauma-recovery/
- *Effects of different core exercises on respiratory parameters ...* https://pmc.ncbi.nlm.nih.gov/articles/PMC4668176/
- *Balance Exercises for Seniors: 11 Moves to Try* https://www.healthline.com/health/exercise-fitness/balance-exercises-for-seniors
- *Mindful Movement: How It's Done and Why It's Good for You* https://www.fitnessblender.com/articles/mindful-movement-how-it-s-done-and-why-it-s-good-for-you
- *Developing Your Own Daily Practice* https://somaticmovementcenter.com/daily-practice/
- *Somatic Awareness: The Science Of Connecting Mind And Body* https://www.brainfirstinstitute.com/blog/somatic-awareness-the-science-of-connecting-mind-and-body#:~:text=Research%20suggests%20that%20enhanced%20somatic,overall%20psychological%20wellbeing%20(14).text=Increased%20somatic%20awareness%20can%20also%20have%20substantial%20benefits%20for%20physical%20health.
- *Somatic Therapy Toolkit - Lisa Powers - Official Site* https://lisapowers.co/somatic-therapy-toolkit/
- *6 Ways to Bust Through a Workout Plateau* https://www.healthline.com/nutrition/workout-plateau
- *The Importance of Mood and Motivation of an Individual in the ...* https://digitalcommons.unl.edu/cgi/viewcontent.cgi?article=153826context=honorstheses
- *Growth beliefs predict exercise efficacy, value and frequency* https://www.sciencedirect.com/science/article/abs/pii/S1469029217306696
- *Community Dojo » Strozzi Institute for Somatics* https://strozziinstitute.org/community-dojo/
- *Holotropic Breathwork Benefits and Risks* https://www.verywellmind.com/holotropic-breathwork-4175431
- *9 Simple Steps to Start Intuitive Exercise* https://www.sarahgoldrd.com/intuitive-exercise/
- *Biofeedback* https://www.mayoclinic.org/tests-procedures/biofeedback/about/pac-20384664
- *Somatic Experiencing for Trauma Recovery* https://www.icanotes.com/2024/03/28/somatic-experiencing-therapy-for-trauma-recovery/
- *Moving With Pain: What Principles From Somatic Practices ...* https://pmc.ncbi.nlm.nih.gov/articles/PMC7868595/
- *How to Improve Athletic Performance with Clinical Somatics* https://essentialsomatics.com/how-to-improve-athletic-performance-with-clinical-

somatics/#:~:text=Clinical%20Somatics%20is%20an%20excellent,or%20knew%20they%20could%20have.

- *The Magic of Somatic Exercise for Women over 50* https://www.fit50andfabulous.com/the-magic-of-somatic-exercise-for-women-over-50/
- *Moving With Pain: What Principles From Somatic Practices ...* https://pmc.ncbi.nlm.nih.gov/articles/PMC7868595/
- *Reflective Practice in Physical Therapy: A Scoping Review* https://pmc.ncbi.nlm.nih.gov/articles/PMC6665949/
- *Somatic Exercises: The Ultimate Guide To Enhancing Your ...* https://www.re-origin.com/articles/somatic-exercises
- *The Pace of the Learning Process* https://somaticmovementcenter.com/pace-learning-process/
- *Somatics Case Studies* https://somatics.org/about/casestudies

www.ingramcontent.com/pod-product-compliance
Lightning Source LLC
Chambersburg PA
CBHW062055270326
41931CB00013B/3089